THE CROWN OF LIFE

ABOUT THE AUTHOR

Kirpal Singh (1894-1974) of Delhi, India began, at a young age, an intense search for a true spiritual Master. For years he investigated the claims of yogis and saints representing many schools of thought. His search culminated in initiation by the great saint of Beas, Baba Sawan Singh. For twenty-four years he diligently studied under his Master's guidance, and was chosen to succeed him in the spiritual line. Thereafter, he served as a spiritual Master for twenty-six years and initiated more than 120,000 disciples throughout the world. He is the author of over twenty books on various aspects of spirituality. In addition, he served as president of the World Fellowship of Religions, and was the organizer of the World Conference on the Unity of Man.

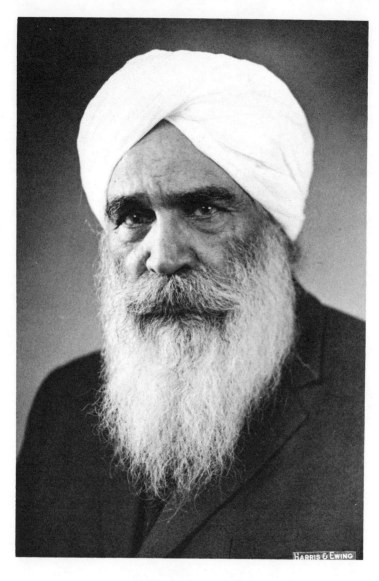

Sant Kirpal Singh Ji
(1894-1974)

THE CROWN OF LIFE

A Study in Yoga

KIRPAL SINGH

SAWAN KIRPAL PUBLICATIONS

Library of Congress Catalog: 79-67543
ISBN 0-918224-09-8

First published by Ruhani Satsang, Delhi, 1961
Second Edition, 1965
Third Edition, 1970
  Second Printing, 1971
  Third Printing, 1973
Fourth Edition published by Sawan Kirpal Publications, 1980
Bowling Green, Virginia 22427, and
2 Canal Road, Vijay Nagar, Delhi-110009, India
  Second Printing, 1985

Printed in the United States of America

Dedicated
to the Almighty God
working through all Masters who have come
and Baba Sawan Singh Ji Maharaj
at whose lotus feet
the writer imbibed sweet elixir of
Holy Naam—the Word

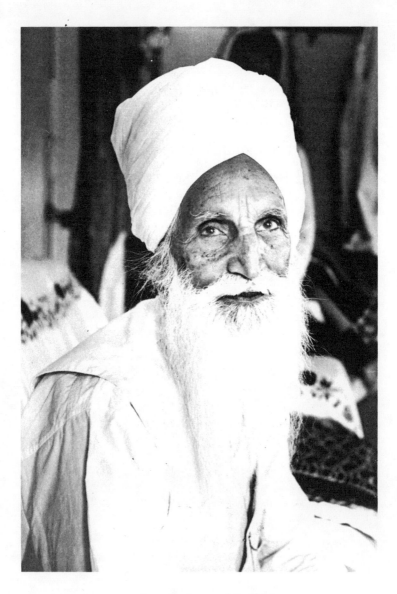

Baba Sawan Singh Ji
(1858-1948)

Preface

THIS study of comparative yoga was initially stimulated by the various queries on the subject which kept pouring in from seekers and disciples in the West. But in trying to answer them in a systematic and comprehensive manner, it has grown into something much larger than its original intent. As it has now evolved it may, I hope, be of service not only to those whose questions first led to its writing, but to all seekers in general who wish to understand what yoga is, the varieties of its forms and their respective modes and spiritual efficacy.

In this age of publishing, there is no dearth of books on yoga. However, if one scrutinizes them carefully, one finds that the majority fall short in one direction or another. They either treat it as primarily a system of *asanas* and physical exercises, or as an abstract and highly monistic system of thought, positing the unity of all existence and the ultimate oneness of the individual soul and the Oversoul. In either case, the view of yoga that we gather is an incomplete one, reducing it from a practical mode of spiritual transcendence and union with the Absolute, to a system of physical culture or school (or group of schools) of philosophy.

To avoid the possibility of such error, the ultimate aim of all yoga, at-one-ment with the Supreme Lord, has been kept as a focusing point for all discussions in this study. All the important forms, ancient and modern, are taken up in turn, their practices explained and discussed, and the extent to which each can lead us toward the final goal evaluated. This last is perhaps the most easily misunderstood and the most widely confused aspect of a comparative study of yoga. It is a characteristic of mystic experience that the soul as it ascends to a plane higher than the one to which it is accustomed, tends (in the absence of superior guidance) to mistake the higher plane as the very highest, the Absolute Realm. And so we find that most yogas, while taking us up to a certain point on the inner journey, mistake this for its end, and for a relative validity claim for themselves an absolute one.

The only way by which we can effectively evaluate the comparative spiritual value of each yogic form and so escape the present state of confusion, is by adopting as our standard the very highest form of yoga, whose potency is absolute and not merely relative. This standard is provided by the *Surat Shabd Yoga* also known as *Sant Mat* (or the path of the *Sants* or Masters of this mystic school), the veritable Crown of Life. By following its practices under proper guidance, its adepts have reached realms not known to other mystic schools, and have finally merged with the Supreme Lord in His Absolute, Nameless and Formless State. They have, in their compositions, repeatedly affirmed the incomparable superiority of this Yoga of the Sound Current and, while describing through direct inner perception the varying spiritual range of other yogas, have gone on to expound the absolute nature of their own.

Once a seeker can begin to grasp the perspectives on comparative mysticism which Sant Mat can provide, he will, I believe, find this extremely complex subject becoming progressively clearer to him. He will see that the contradictions which disturb so many when they first undertake a comparative study of mysticism are not essential to mystic experience as such, but are the result of a confusion of a relative truth with an absolute one, an error which does not exist for those, who by following the highest path, have experienced first-hand all the inner states, and know the points up to which each yoga can lead. He will no longer be tempted to evade the issue of spirituality by dismissing it as a mere remnant of old superstition and black magic but will begin to see it as a kind of timeless inner science with its own unchanging laws and varying modes of operation, with knowledge which is not static, but has developed as men have moved from lower to higher forms of yoga. And above all, he will, I hope, realize that mergence with the Supreme Lord is no mere day-dream or hypothetical postulate of a monistic school of philosophy, but a living possibility whose realization is the true end of human existence and whose attainment, given the right guidance, the right method and the right effort, lies within the reach of all, irrespective of age, sex, race or creed.

Sawan Ashram, Delhi   KIRPAL SINGH

June 6, 1961

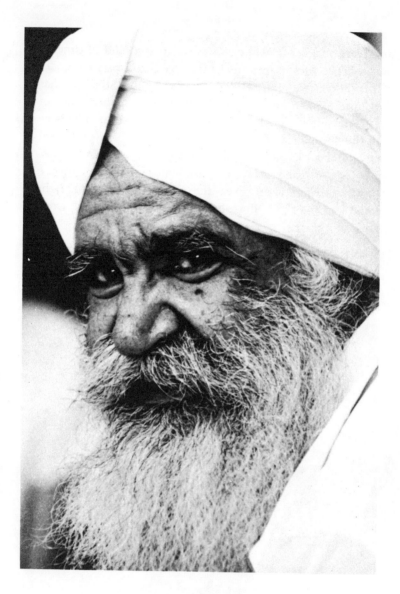

Living Master
Sant Darshan Singh Ji

Table of Contents

PART TWO

The Study of Surat Shabd Yoga

Charts

PART ONE

The Yogic Patterns

CHAPTER ONE

Yoga: An Introduction

ALL the great teachers of humanity, at all times and in all climes—the Vedic Rishis, Zoroaster, Mahavira, Buddha, Christ, Mohammed, Nanak, Kabir, Baba Farid, Hazrat Bahu, Shamas Tabrez, Maulana Rumi, Tulsi Sahib, Swamiji and many others—gave to the world but one *sadhna* or spiritual discipline. As God is one, the God-way too cannot but be one. The true religion or the way back to God is of God's own making and hence it is the most ancient as well as the most natural way, with no artifice or artificiality about it. In its practical working, the system needs the guidance of an adept or a teacher well versed in the theory and practice of *Para Vidya,* the Science of the Beyond, as it is called, for it lies beyond the grasp of the mind and of the sense-faculties. Where the world's philosophies end, there the true religion starts. The scriptural texts give us, at best, some account of the Path so far as it can be put into imperfect words, but cannot take us to the Path nor can they guide us on the Path.

The spiritual Path is essentially a practical Path. It is only the spirit—disencumbered and depersonalized—that can undertake the spiritual journey. The inner man, the soul in man, has to rise above body-consciousness before it can traverse into higher consciousness or the consciousness of the cosmos and of the beyond. All this and more becomes possible through the *Surat Shabd Yoga* or the union of "self" in man (*Surat* or consciousness) with the *Shabd* or Sound Principle, through the grace of some Master-soul.

3

In order to have a clear idea of the teachings of the Masters from the hoary past right to the present time, it would be worth our while to study the nature and extent of the Surat Shabd Yoga and its teachings in relation to the various yogic systems as taught by the ancients, and also the principles of Advaitism as propounded by Shankaracharya.

The term *yoga* is derived from the Sanskrit root *yuj* which means meeting, union, communion, consummation, abstraction, realization, absorption or metaphysical philosophizing of the highest type, that promises to bring close proximity between the soul and the Oversoul (*jiva-atma* and *Parmatma* or *Brahman*). Patanjali, the reputed father of the yoga system, after the fashion of his progenitor Gaudapada, defines yoga as elimination of the *vritis* or modulations that always keep surging in the mind-stuff or *chit* in the form of ripples. He calls it *chit vriti nirodha* or the supression of the vritis, i.e., clearing the mind of the mental oscillations. According to Yajnavalkya, yoga means to effect, or to bring about, at-one-ment of the individual soul with Ishwar or Brahman. The yogins generally define it as the unfoldment of the spirit from and disrobing it of the numerous enshrouding sheaths in which it is enveloped in its physical existence. *Sant Mat* or the Path of the Masters, far from denying any of these objectives of yoga, accepts and endorses in full all that is said above and, in some measure, agrees to the aims and ends thereof, but regards them at best as mere pointers to the goal. It does not rest there, however, but goes beyond and tells us of the "Way Out" of the mighty maze of the universe and the "Way In" to the Heavenly Home of the Father, the spiritual journey that the spirit has to undertake from death to life immortal (*Fana* to *Baqa*), by rising above body-consciousness by means of a regular system of self-analysis and withdrawal of the spirit currents from the body and concentrating them at the seat of the soul (*Tisra Til*), and then gradually passing through the intermediary centers beyond *Bunk-naal,* the inverted, tube-like passage, until it reaches the final stage of consummation and attains at-one-ment with its Source.

Here one might ask the question as to the need for union between the soul and the Oversoul, when the two are essentially the same and are already embedded one in the other. Theoretically speaking, this is correct, but how many of us are consciously aware of this and work practically in the light and life of this knowledge and awareness? On the other hand, the soul is always following the lead of the mind, the mind that of the senses, and the senses that of the sense-objects, with the result that the soul, by constant association with the mind and the senses for ages upon ages, has completely lost its own individual (undivided) identity and has for all practical purposes become identified with the mind. It is this veil of ignorance which has come in between the soul and the Oversoul that has to be removed to enable the soul to come into its own, to realize its inherent nature and then to seek its real home and gain life eternal. All religions were originally designed by man solely with this end in view but unfortunately in the course of time man gradually drifts away from reality and becomes the slave of his own handicrafts and religions, as religions deteriorate into institutionalized churches and temples, rigid codes of moral and social conduct, lacking the living touch and the pulsating life-impulse of their founders.

"I know no disease of the soul but ignorance," says Ben Jonson. How to remove the veil of ignorance is the problem of problems. We have allowed it to grow into an impervious rock too hard to be blasted. Still, the sages have provided various means to rend the otherwise impenetrable veil, such as *Jnana Yoga, Bhakti Yoga* and *Karma Yoga* and other methods. The light of true knowledge, as visualized by Jnana Yoga, may be able to dispel the darkness of ignorance, just as a lighted candle may dispel darkness from a dark room. By Bhakti Yoga one may be able to change the course of hatred, separateness and duality into that of love for all, at-one-ment and oneness with all living creatures and thereby be established in the all-embracing love for all. Finally, by means of Karma Yoga one may be able to root out feelings of selfishness, egocentricity, self-aggrandizement and self-love and engage in charitable deeds of philanthropy and similar activities, which may be beneficial to mankind in general, and acquire fellow feelings and love for all, see the reflex of the universe within his own self and that of his self in all others, and realize ultimately the principle of the Fatherhood of God and the brotherhood of man. These are, in the main, the three paths, or rather three aspects of an integrated path of head, heart and hand, whereby one may achieve the desired end, the union of the soul with the Oversoul. They may for convenience be briefly termed the process of self-mastery, self-sublimation and self-sacrifice, leading ultimately to "Cosmic Consciousness," or awareness of the all-pervading Reality as the basis of all that exists.

The objective in each case is the same and each aims at the same target, though in the initial elementary stages each of them starts from dualistic considerations. It is from dualism that one starts, and in non-dualism (advaitism) that one ends; and for this one may take to the path of divine knowledge, of universal love and devotion or of selfless service of humanity.

> The target ever remains the same,
> Though the archers aiming at it be so many.
>
> RAJAB

In Jnana Yoga, for instance, one has to develop the faculty of discrimination, so as to be able to distinguish between *agyan* and *gyan*, i.e., ignorance and true knowledge, the illusory character of Maya and the reality of Brahman. When he is con-

vinced of the latter he gets glimpses of nothing but Brahman
pervading everywhere in Its limitless essence, immanent in all
forms and colors which take their design and hue from that
essence alone. This perception is the dawning of true knowledge and divine wisdom.

In Bhakti Yoga, likewise, we begin with the twin principles
of *Bhagat* and *Bhagwant,* or the devotee and the deity, and
the devotee gradually loses his little self and sees his deity all-
pervading, and his own self expands so as to embrace the
totality as does his own *Isht-deva.* "Whoever enters a salt
mine, tends to become salt." As you think, so you become.

Again, in Karma Yoga, one may enter the *Karma Kshetra*
or the field of actions, under some impelling force to begin
with, but in course of time he learns the value of selfless
Karma. Karmas when performed for their own sake without
any attachment to the fruit thereof, cease to be binding, and
by force of habit one gradually becomes *Neh Karma* (action-
less in action), or a still point in the ever-revolving wheel of
life. In this way, when one from the circumference of his
being reaches the center of his being, he acquires inaction in
action and is freed from the binding effect of Karmas.

Vritis: What they are

When a current emanating from the spirit strikes any object, such as a physical thing, a mental feeling, an idea, or a
sensory sensation, and returns to its source, it is called a *vriti.*
The vriti produces a modulation in the mind-stuff. All our
knowledge of the world without and within comes from vritis
or the rays of thought. A ray of light, reflected from or originating from an object, passes through the eyes to the brain,
where it is converted into thought impressions making us
aware of the object.

Vritis are of five kinds:

(i) *Parman*: The relationship between the pure soul and

Prakriti or Nature is called Parman. In every manifestation, the pure soul finds its own essence at the core and nothing is apart and distinct from It.

(ii) *Vipreh*: The relationship between the knowing soul and Prakriti or Nature's object is called Vipreh. It takes in and accepts the manifested form as it is, but remains sceptical of the one and active life-principle at the core of it.

(iii) *Vikalp*: It is the relationship that the mind-ridden soul has with the objects, producing doubt and delusion as to the objects themselves, their existence, their intrinsic nature and the life-essence at their core.

(iv) *Nidra*: It is the relationship that the prana-covered soul has with the objects. It embraces in its fold the twin states of dream and deep slumber, regardless of the existing surroundings.

(v) *Smriti*: It is the relationship of the embodied soul with the objects of the world on the physical plane.

All these vritis constitute so many hurdles in the way of the soul seeking to understand its true and essential nature, which in reality is nothing but that of God. Kabir therefore says: "Soul is of the same essence as that of God."

Similarly, the Muslim divines express the same idea when they speak of the soul as *Amar-i-Rabbi* or the fiat of God.

If one could but clear the *chit* of the vritis (*chit vriti nirodha,* as it is called), nothing would be left except the pure essence of Godhead. Hence we have the oft-repeated famous dicta on yoga, as in the following:

> *Chit-vriti nirodha (clearing the mind of the mental oscillations) is the essence of yoga.*
>
> PANTANJALI

> *At-one-ment of the soul and the Oversoul is yoga.*
>
> YAJNAVALKYA

*Extrication of the soul from the materials of life by
disrobing it of the enshrouding sheaths, is yoga.*

MACHHANDRA NATH AND GORAKH NATH

The easiest, the most ancient, and the most natural way to
gain the fruits of yoga, as taught by Kabir, Nanak and others
before and after them, is that of Shabd Yoga or Sehaj Yoga,
as given by all the Master saints from time immemorial.
When the spirit is able, by practice of the spiritual *sadhna,* to
cast off, one by one, the various coverings, it becomes a pure
spirit, complete in itself, a conscious entity, self-existent and
self-luminous, ever the same and eternally free. According to
the saints, yoga is communion of the soul with the holy Word
(God into expression), the power of God or the spirit of God:
*Sruti, Sraosha, Kalma, Naam** or the Holy Spirit as variously
designated by the various sages each in his own particular
time.

Soul and Oversoul

1. Soul is the Reality and the Essence. It is one as well as
a totality. In one there is always the delusion of many, and the
totality does signify the existence therein of so many parts. The
ideas of a part and of the whole go cheek by jowl, and both
the part as well as the whole are characterized by the similar-
ity of the essential nature in them.

2. The essence of a thing has its own attributive nature and
the two cannot be separated from each other. Just as the essence is both one and many, so is the case with its attributive
nature.

3. The essence of a thing is its *Johar,* its very life breath.
It is the only primal principle that pervades everywhere and is

---

* For detailed explanation of these terms, please refer to the book
Naam or Word by the same author.

the reality behind all forms and colors. This active life principle is the very source of creation and goes variously by the names of Prakriti in the subtle, Pradhan in the causal, and Maya or matter in the physical world.

4. The attributive nature of a thing is its integrated part and parcel in which its nature inheres. Just take the case of light. Can light be conceived of as apart from the sun, or radiant vitality apart from a gloriously healthy personality? One does not exist without the other as the two are inseparable and fully embedded in each other.

5. Any attempt to consider the two—nature and its essence—as separate, even if only in imagination, is bound to bring in the idea of duality. It is only in terms of this duality that one can conceive of the creation as distinct from the creative principle as being the result of the outer play of the twin forces of spirit, called matter and soul. The scientific investigations too have now come to the irresistible conclusion that all life is one continuous existence at different levels and what we call inert matter is nothing but energy at its lowest stage.

In Nature itself, both in the subtle and causal planes, these two principles are always at work: God and Prakriti in the subtle, God and Pradhan in the causal, and soul and matter in the physical universe. The creation everywhere is but the outcome of the impact of the one on the other.

6. Soul then is the life-principle and the root cause at the core of everything, for nothing can come into manifestation without it. It has a quickening effect, and imparts its life-impulse to the seemingly inert matter by contact with it. It is by the life and light of the quickening impulse of the soul that matter assumes so many forms and colors with their variety of patterns and designs which we see in the Universe.

7. This life current or soul is extremely subtle, a self effulgent spark of Divine Light, a drop from the Ocean of Consciousness, with no beginning and no end, and eternally the

same, an unchangeable permanence, boundless, complete in Itself, an ever-existent and all-sentient entity, immanent in every form, visible and invisible, for all things manifest themselves because of It. Nothing is made that is not made by It.

The One remains, the many change and pass,
Life like a dome of many-colored glass,
Stains the white radiance of Eternity.

SHELLEY

8. Just as the sun spreads out its rays in the world, as an ocean carries on its surface bubbles, ripples, waves, tides and currents, and as a forest is made up of innumerable trees, so does Oversoul or God, when looked at through His creation, appear to be split into so many forms, exhibiting and reflecting the light and life of God in a rich panorama of variegated colors. Yet His spirit runs through all alike, just as a string through so many beads, while He, unconcerned, remains apart from all in His own fullness.

9. The first downward projection of the spiritual current, as it emanated from God, brought into manifestation ether (*akash*), which is the most subtle of the elements and spreads everywhere in space. This has two aspects. One is that of the spirit or soul remaining unmanifest in the ether, and the other that of the manifest ether, wherein the two forces, positive and negative, which are inherent in it, further combined and brought into manifestation air (*vayu*) and exactly in the same way the manifest air gave birth to fire (*agni*) and the manifest fire produced water (*jal*) and the manifest water led to the formation of earth (*prithvi*), while the spirit of each element which is essentially the same remained unmanifest throughout.

In the same way as above, what we call God has an essential Godhood, absolute and imageless, the life and spirit of the Universe, and at the same time the Universe itself with its varied creations full of and manifesting so many forms and colors, appearing and disappearing like ripples in the sea of life. The unmanifest and impersonal God is free from all attributes, while His individualized rays, as manifested in countless forms and colors by constant contact with Maya, Prakriti and Pradhan (physical, subtle and causal) feel themselves, through ignorance of their true nature, as limited and separate from each other and are thereby drawn into the ambit of the inexorable Karmic Law or the Law of Cause and Effect, which entails a consequence for every deed, every word and every thought. What is unfulfilled in one life is fulfilled in another, and thus the giant wheel of life and death once set in motion goes on perpetually by the force of its own inexhaustible momentum. Herein lies the difference between the individualized soul on the one hand, and the Great Soul of the Universe (called God) on the other, the one being bound and limited, the other being without bounds or limits.

Prakriti or matter

The term *Prakriti* is a compound term and is derived from the Sanskrit root *pra* meaning "first," and *kar* signifying "to act" and thus *Prakriti* stands for "original matter" (latent energy) which, when acted upon by positive spirit force, brings into being the many forms, patterns and designs in the vast creation of the Great Creator. This is called *Maya,* and all that can be seen or felt by any of the senses falls in the category of matter or *Prakriti*. Matter, as explained above, is latent energy at its lowest level, which is quickened into activity (activated) and made to assume the many different forms that we perceive as patent. This process from passivity into activity of energy leads to creation, or manifestation of the hitherto unmanifested spirit force.

Brahman or spirit force comes into being only through a gross covering (*kaya*).

Just as the totality of the seemingly individualized souls goes to make Oversoul (God), so also the mighty maze of the created beings and things with different forms and colors in their totality, is called Prakriti.

Prakriti by itself can neither be felt by the senses nor has it any existence of itself, but comes into manifestation only when acted upon by the spirit force. Just as the rays of the sun have no existence apart from the sun and appear only when the sun rises on the horizon, so does Prakriti, in conjunction with the life-impulse, assume innumerable shapes and forms beyond the human ken, and the One invisible soul seems to get diversified into individualized parts, with different names and varied species that baffle description and solution. Still, the yogins have taken into account the five *koshas* or the enshrouding sheaths that have come to cover up the spirit current in its downward descent, and have devised and formulated ways and means to remove them. These koshas or coverings may briefly be described as:

1. *Vigyan-mai Kosh*: Covering of the mental apparatus or intellect with its two phases: one concerned with knowledge (*gyan*) on the physical plane and the other with enlightenment (*vigyan*) on the spiritual planes. This is the first covering in which the spirit gets wrapped as it comes in contact with the subtle matter called Prakriti. The light of the soul, as it reflects in the intellectual center, brings into motion what is commonly known as intellect, consisting of inner spiritual perception and outer cognition. The soul, along with this reflected intellectual ability, becomes both cognitive and perceptive.

2. *Man-o-mai Kosh*: This is the second covering or sheath that the intellectualized or the cognitive soul wraps around itself by further intensive contact with Prakriti, which now begins to reflect the mind-stuff as well; and with this added faculty the soul becomes inclined toward the mind and gradually gets mind-ridden.

3. *Pran-mai Kosh*: The covering of the *pranas* (the vital airs) constitutes the third sheath around the soul. As the thinking (cognitive) and mind-bound soul presses still further upon Prakriti (matter), it begins to vibrate with pranas, which are of ten types according to their different functions. This makes the cognitive and mind-bound soul to be *pran-mai,* or impelled by a quickening effect.

4. *Anna-mai Kosh*: When the cognitive, mind-bound and impulsive soul works upon the Prakriti, it forges therein yet another type of covering, that of *anna-mai.* This is the last of the five sheaths, and for its maintenance it begins to feel a continuing need for *anna* or foodstuff, and other sense objects.

This anna-mai covering is just an inner lining of the physical body (gross matter), which in fact is its outer manifestation; and it continues to wrap the soul even when its outer form, i.e., body, declines, decays and disintegrates.

The existence of this coarse physical body depends upon the healthy condition of the Anna-mai Kosh on the inside of it.

Some of the souls, even when they cast off the outer physical body, still hanker after food because of the Anna-mai Kosh, hunt after the pleasures of the world and continue to haunt human habitations in their wanderings for satisfaction of their innate cravings. It is to satisfy these cravings of the physically disembodied souls that the Hindus perform *pind dan* and *saradhs,* and make propitiatory offerings to the *manes* or the departed souls so that they may find rest and peace.

5. However, it is *Anand-mai Kosh* (Bliss) that is the first and the foremost of these Koshas or coverings. This is almost an integral part of the soul itself. It is the most subtle sheath, like that of a thin covering over a lighted candelabra. One experiences it a little when in deep and dreamless slumber (*sushupti*), for on waking up he retains a hazy idea of the *anand* or bliss that he experienced in that completely undisturbed state of rest.

These then are the five koshas or *hijabs* (curtains or covering mantles) as the Muslims call them, and they cover the soul, fold within fold. The aim or purpose of all yogas is to gradually disentangle the soul from these coverings one by one, until it is finally disengaged from all of them and is restored to its original and pristine glorious state of self luminosity (*Swayam Jyoti*), which is no less than that of several suns put together. This is the stage of *Aham Brahm Asmi* or "I am Brahm," and when attained, one not only feels himself to be at oneness with God, but actually hails God with the words—*Ayam Athma Brahma*—"O God! I am of the same essence as Thou art." Most of the yoga systems take this to be the be-all and end-all of all spiritual endeavors. This in fact is the highest and the last stage of self-realization, but is yet a halfway house on the spiritual journey—a stage of no mean consequence, for it is from here that a rare soul starts toward the much coveted goal of complete realization of God, since it is *Khud Shanasi* (Self-knowledge) that gradually leads on to *Khuda Shanasi* (knowledge of God).

Self-knowledge and actual self-realization is the culminating point in the process of self-analysis, without which one cannot proceed Godward and enter into the Kingdom of God. In this process of inversion and withdrawal of the spirit within by rising above body-consciousness and freeing the spirit from the tentacles of the body and mind, the easiest, quickest, and surest process is by communion with the *Shabd* or the Sound Current (the Holy Word), and this is the only means for God-realization. It is the most ancient way the world has known, coming down as it does from the dawn of creation itself. It is coeval with Man from the day he became separated from his Father in Heaven. All the great Masters of mankind gave this Word to their disciples. This is baptism with the Holy Spirit, as Christ put it.

Relationship between the three bodies and the five koshas

The human body consists of three raiments: physical, astral or subtle, and the causal or seed-body.

In the physical body we have all the five koshas or coverings, and this is why we, in our waking state, get some knowledge and experience of all the five things: bliss, cognition (inner or outer), mindfulness (*chit* and its *vritis* or mental modulations), pranic vibrations and the physical system.

As one rises into the astral or the subtle body, one loses consciousness of the physical existence, while the soul mentally experiences the rest of the four states, viz., bliss, cognition, mindfulness and pranic vibrations.

As the spirit travels higher on into the causal body, even the mental apparatus itself drops off and only the power of *smriti* (remembrance) remains, and it witnesses and gives an account of the bliss experienced in that state.

Division of creation according to the koshas

All beings from gods to man, as well as the other forms of life, including plants, are classified into five categories in relation to the preponderance of one or the other of the faculties:

1. Purely cognitive beings, like Brahma, Vishnu and Mahesh, etc.
2. Beings endowed with mind-stuff: Indra and other deities, gods and goddesses, etc.
3. Beings endowed with pranic vibrations: *Yakshas, Gandharbas* and other spirits, etc.
4. Physical beings: Men, animals, birds, reptiles and insects, etc.

The creatures endowed with physical bodies have all the five koshas or coverings in them in varying degrees of density

(Anand-mai, Vigyan-mai, Mano-mai, Pran-mai and Anna-mai); while those endowed with pranic vibrations have but four koshas, dropping off Anna-mai. Similarly, creatures gifted with the mind-stuff have but three, dropping off Pran-mai as well, and again, cognitive beings have but two, namely Anand-mai and Vigyan-mai, as they are freed from the shackles of the mind, the pranas and the need for anna or foodstuff.

There is thus a very close correspondence between the five primary elements (earth, water, fire, air and ether), of which the bodies are made, and the koshas or coverings. In fact, the koshas themselves are, more or less, the effective result of the five basic elements and endow creatures with the five faculties enumerated above.

5. The liberated soul (*jivan mukta*) has but a transparent veil of Anand-mai Kosh. Spirit in its pure and unalloyed form is the creator, for all creation springs from it, and is sometimes known as *Shabd Brahm*. It is the self-effulgent light, self-existent, and the causeless cause of everything visible and invisible. The spirit and God both are alike in their nature and essence, i.e., subtlety and bliss. This blissfulness is the very first offspring of the interaction of soul and Prakriti, and being the primal manifestation of the Godhood in the soul, remains the longest to the end in its fullness in spite of the other four coverings enveloping it and bedimming its luster. Blissfulness being the essential and inseparable quality of the soul inheres in its very nature. This is why the searching soul ever feels restless, and feels terribly the loss of its essence in the mighty swirl of the world. This is why Christ emphatically declared:

> *Take heed that the light which is in thee be not darkness.*

ST. LUKE

Having thus lost sight of the inner bliss, we try to find happiness in the worldly objects and take momentary pleasures as a synonym for true happiness but very soon get disillusioned. This leads to the innate quest for real happiness. It is the eternal quest in the human breast, and from outward, ephemeral and evanescent pleasures one is forced to turn inwards in search of true happiness. This leads on to the beginning of the various yoga systems, one and all, according to the needs of the individual aspirants.

1. Persons with gross tendencies, animal instincts, and interested only in body-building processes and developing the Anna-mai Atma, successfully take recourse to Hatha Yoga.

2. Persons afflicted with wind or gastric troubles, due to obsessions with *pran vayu* in their system, can combat these with the help of Pran Yoga.

3. Persons with Mano-mai Atma in the ascendant, and suffering from *mal, avaran* and *vikshep,* i.e., mental impurities, ignorance and modulations of the mind, can with the help of Raja Yoga conquer and pierce through the Mano-mai Kosh.

4. Persons gifted with a strong intellectual bent of mind are ever engaged in finding the why and wherefore of things. Such aspirants take to the path of *Vigyan* or Jnana Yoga.

5. Those who are anxious to escape from the world and all that is worldly and seek bliss for its own sake have the path of Anand Yoga or the yoga of True Happiness, called the Sehaj Yoga.

In the Sehaj Yoga, the aspirant does not have to undergo any of the rigorous disciplines characteristic of the other yogas. He must have a sincere and ceaseless yearning for the end of all ends, the goal of all goals, not content with a mere mastery of his physical and mental powers. And when there is such a longing, sooner or later he would find, as Ramakrishna found Totapuri, an adept to put him in touch with the vital life current within, and the current by its own force and attraction will draw him up without any excessive struggle or effort on his part. It is this that makes it in a sense the easiest of all yogas and thus it is often called Sehaj Yoga (the effortless yoga). It can be practised with equal ease by a child as well by an old man; by a woman as well as a man; by the intellectually gifted and ingenious as well as the simple hearted; by the sanyasin as well as the householder. It consists in attuning the soul to the spiritual current ever vibrating within, hence it is known as the Surat Shabd Yoga, or the Yoga of the Sound Current.

With these preliminary remarks, we are now in a position to discuss the subject of yoga with its various essentials as taught by Patanjali, to understand the part that each plays, the technique involved therein, how each step works out, and how far the yogic exercises help practically in achieving the desired result—liberation of soul from the bondage of mind and matter—so as to realize its own potential nature as distinct from body-consciousness, and then to rise into Cosmic Consciousness and further on into Super-Cosmic Consciousness. It is the freed soul that has to experience "awareness" at varying levels, from realization of the "self" to that of "Cosmic" and ultimately to that of "Super-Cosmic" or God.

CHAPTER TWO

Yog Vidya and Yog Sadhna

The Path of Yoga in Theory and Practice

1. The Basis of Ancient Yoga

Origin and technique of the yoga system

FROM the *Yajnavalkya Smriti,* we learn that Hiranyagarbha
(Brahma) was the original teacher of yoga. But the yoga
system, as a system, was first expounded by Patanjali, the
great thinker and philosopher, in his *Yoga Sutras,* sometime
before the Christian era. The yogic system is one of the six
schools of Indian philosophy (*Khat Shastras*) that were sys-
tematized and developed to set in order Indian thought
concerning the cosmos, the individual soul, and their inter-
relation. These philosophies resulted from an attempt at refor-
mation and restoration of the ancient and time-honored
concepts on psychological and metaphysical matters.

The word *yoga* in common parlance means "method." In
its technical sense, it connotes "yoking" or "union" of the individual soul with the Oversoul or God. The English word
"yoke" signifies "to unite" or "join together" and "to place
oneself under yoke" (discipline). In this context, the yoga
system denotes a "methodical discipline," which aims on the
one hand at *viyog* (unyoking), or separation of the individualized soul from mind and matter, and on the other hand, *yog,*
or yoking it with Brahman. It, therefore, means and implies
the search for the transcendental and the divine in man, or to

find the "noumenal" in the "phenomenal" by reducing the physical and metaphysical states to their most essential common factor, the basis and the substratum of all that exists, whether visible or invisible. As such, yogic methods imply a system of mighty effort, most strenuous endeavour and hard striving to attain perfection through the control of the physical body, the ever-active mind, the self-assertive ego or will, the searching and questioning intellect, the pranic vibrations, the restless faculties and powerful senses. Allegorically, the present state of the individualized soul is described as riding in the chariot of the body, with dazed intellect as the charioteer, the infatuated mind as the reins, and the senses as the powerful steeds rushing headlong into the field of sense objects and sense pleasures. All this goes to show that a student of yoga discipline has to undertake a course of an extremely strict and ordered activity as may help to depersonalize the soul and free it from all the limiting adjuncts of life, physical, mental and supramental, and then to contact it with the power of God and achieve union with God.

The word *yoga* is however not to be confused with *yog-maya* and "yogic powers" which denote respectively, the supreme Power of God per se (creating, controlling and sustaining the entire creation), and the psychic powers (*Ridhis* and *Siddhis*) that one may acquire on the path of yoga. Again, *yog vidya* or the science of yoga has a two-fold aspect; the physical as well as the spiritual. In the former sense, it has come to mean a yogic system of physical culture aiming at an all-around development of the various component parts of the human body. But we are concerned here with the spiritual aspect of yoga that aims at the well-being of the spirit or soul, the real life-principle in man, at present neglected and ignored. The term *yoga* in this context is, therefore, to be strictly confined to one of the systems of philosophic thought as derived from the Vedas, and is concerned with the sole object

of regaining the soul (through spiritual discipline), now lost
in the activity of mind and matter, with which it has come to
identify itself by long and constant association for aeons upon
aeons. Yoga, in brief, stands for a technique of reorientation
and reintegration of the spirit in man, the lost continent of
his true self.

Fundamental concepts

Yoga presupposes two factors that account for the creation
of the world: (1) *Ishwar* or God and (2) *Avidya* or Maya.
While the former is all intelligent, the latter is altogether unin-
telligent. Man too is a combination of these two basic principles. *Jiva* or the individual soul though intrinsically of the
same essence as that of God, is encased in mind and matter.
The soul, conditioned as it is in the time-space-cause world,
has but an imperfect perception and cannot see the reality,
the *atman* or the Divine Ground, in which it rests and from
where it gets its luminosity. While *antahkaran,* or the mind, is
the reflector, the atman is the illuminator, the light of which
is reflected through the senses that perceive the world. The
world then is the conjunction of the "seer" and the "seen."
The detachment of this conjunction is the escape, and perfect
insight is the means of escape. Salvation therefore lies in the
isolation of the seer from the seen, the complete detachment
of the subjective from all that is objective: physical, mental,
and causal, so that the "Self" which is the seer, may see itself
in its own luminosity or "Light of the Void," as it is called.

To free the individual soul from the shackles of mind and
matter, yoga insists on (1) concentration, (2) active effort or
striving, which involves the performance of devotional exercises and mental discipline. The highest form of matter is *chit,*
the unfathomable lake of subliminal impressions, and yoga
aims at freeing the inner man or spirit from these fetters. It is
the finest and rarefied principle in matter that constitutes chit

or the little self (ego) in man. Though in itself, it is essentially unconscious, it is subject to modifications by the operation of the three-fold *gunas*. It has also the capacity to contract and expand according to the nature of the body in which it is lodged from time to time, or according to the surrounding circumstances.

This *chit* or mind, though apparently bounded in each individual, is in fact a part of the all-pervading universal mind. The yoga systems aim at transforming the limited and conditioned mind into limitless and unconditioned Universal mind, by developing the *satva* (pure) and by subduing the *rajas* (active) and *tamas* (dense) gunas. In this state, yogins acquire omniscience, being one with the Universal mind (*Brahmandi* or *Nij manas*). Chit is the reflecting mirror for the soul, and exists for *chaitanmaya*, or matter quickened by soul, which is self-luminous and in whose spiritual light takes place all perception, including the light of knowledge, mental and supramental. The subliminal impressions in the chit cause desires and interest, which in turn produce potencies, and these lead to personality, thus setting the wheel of the world in perpetual motion. When once the soul is freed from the *chit, manas, budhi,* and *ahankar,* it comes into its own, and becomes passionless and depersonalized. This is the great deliverance which yoga promises to yogins. At this severance from the four-fold fetters of the mind, the embodied soul (*jiva*) becomes a freed soul (*atman*), unindividualized, self-luminous, and attains realization as such. "Self-realization" then is the highest aim of yoga.

2. The Path and the Branches of Ashtang Yoga

The yogic art is long, tortuous and arduous. The reality of the self lies buried under the debris of the mind, consisting of *mal, avaran* and *vikshep,* viz., filth or impurities, ignorance of the true values of life, and constant vacillations or modulations in the chit. The mental stratum has therefore to be cleared of all these and then to be pierced through and penetrated to find the divine nature of the self or *atman*. To achieve this, one has to conquer desires, to develop steadiness of thought, to cultivate virtues like continence, abstinence, temperance, righteousness, etc., and to develop *vairagya*, or detachment.

To overcome the hindrances and to realize the self, Patanjali gives an elaborate account of what he terms *Ashtang Yoga*, prescribing an eight-fold method consisting of: (1) *Yama*, (2) *Niyama*, (3) *Asana*, (4) *Pranayam*, (5) *Pratyahara*, (6) *Dharna*, (7) *Dhyan* and (8) *Samadhi*.

I - II. YAMAS AND NIYAMAS

Yama: The term *yama* literally means to expel, to eject, to throw out or to eliminate. It denotes abstention from vices and from entertaining any evil thoughts, or accepting any negative impressions which may tend to weaken the mind and the will.

Niyama: The term *niyama* on the contrary, signifies acceptance, cultivation, observance and development of positive virtues, harboring good feelings, and absorbing these virtues into one's system.

Thus, these two words connote the simultaneous rejection of evil, and the assiduous cultivation and acceptance of good, respectively. Patanjali emumerates these abstinences and observances as *ahimsa* (non-injury), *satya* (non-lying), *asteya* (non-stealing), *brahmcharya* (non-sexuality) and *aprigreha* (non-covetousness or non-possessiveness).

In respect of abstinences, it is said:
(i) One who is rooted in *ahimsa*, has no enemies.
(ii) One who is anchored in *satya*, his words cannot but come true and bear fruit.

Some Yamas and Niyamas

YAMAS	NIYAMAS
Abstention from	*Acceptance and observance of*
1 Negation of God.	Faith in God and Godly power.
2 Self-indulgence.	Self-control and chastity (*Brahmcharya* or purity in thoughts, words and deeds).
3 Dishonest and fraudulent livelihood.	Earning a living by honest and truthful means.
4 Unhygienic and impure conditions of life, both within and without.	Cleanliness: inner, by water irrigation within and oxygenation, etc., and outer, by regular skin-baths, hip-baths, sun and air-baths, etc., and hygienic living conditions in sanitary surroundings.
5 Injuring others by thoughts, words and deeds (*himsa*).	Non-injury by thoughts, words and deeds (*ahimsa*).
6 Practicing falsehood, deceit and covetousness.	Cultivating truth, sincerity and charity.
7 Impatience, avarice and selfishness.	Patience, contentment and selfless service.
8 Self-assertion and ego-centricity.	Humility and self-surrender.

(iii) One who is established in *asteya,* is a true friend of nature, and nature lays bare unto him all her riches.

(iv) One who practises *brahmcharya* comes to acquire absolute power.

(v) One who practises *aprigreha,* solves the enigma of life, and to him the past, the present, and the future appear like an open book.

The five observances are: *Shaucha* (purity of body and mind), *Santosh* (contentment), *Tapas* (austerity), *Svadhyaya* (scriptural study including *japa,* etc.) and *Prasadhna* or *Ishvara Pranidhana* (thoughts attuned with, and absolute dependence on, God).

(a) *Shaucha* brings in cleanliness and dislike for *Sparsha* (contact with another's body).

(b) *Santosh* makes one contented and thus mentally rich.

(c) *Tapas* rids one of all impurities and confers supernatural powers (e.g., to atomize oneself, to lose all weight, to become all speed, to gain instantaneous access to any place, to have all wishes fulfilled, to become all-pervasive, to acquire divine powers, to control all beings and elements in nature, etc.). All these come of themselves by contemplating and concentrating on the opposite of what one actually desires.

(d) *Svadhyaya* personifies the deity worshipped.

(e) *Ishvara Pranidhana* brings in satiety and desirelessness.

In the Upanishads, however, each of these lists consists of ten abstinences and observances. Thus *aprigreha* in the first category has given place to kindness, rectitude, forgiveness, endurance, temperance and purity. Similarly, in the second list, *shaucha* has been replaced by faith, charity, modesty, intelligence, *japa* and fasts. However, the end in either case is *sadachar* or righteous living, which prepares the way for

inner spiritual development. The lists of the virtues to be in-
culcated and the vices to be discarded may vary from teacher
to teacher but the pupose is ever the same. Thus, Manu
explains the principles of *sadachar* or *dharma* in terms of his
own categories.

The practice of both yamas and niyamas — restraints and
observances — make up *sadachar* or right conduct, which
constitutes the bedrock of all the religions of the world.
Manu gives us the essence of dharma as *ahimsa, satya, steyam,
shaucham, indriya nigreha* (harmlessness, truthfulness, purity,
right living and control of senses).

According to Sandalya Rishi, the list comprises:

(a) *Shaucha* (external bodily purity along with that of
    place and direction, and internal purity of thoughts,
    feelings and emotions).

(b) *Daya* (mercy and compassion for all living creatures
    in all circumstances).

(c) *Arjava* (balanced and steady mind in all actions and
    under all conditions).

(d) *Dhriti* (fortitude and endurance in all circumstances).

(e) *Mit-ahara* (disciplined life of temperance generally,
    and in foods and drinks in particular).

In the *Bhagavad Gita* too, Lord Krishna lays great stress
on the practice of yamas and niyamas.

The compassionate Buddha also prescribed for his followers
the noble Eight-fold Path of Righteousness, comprising right
views (knowledge), right aspirations (determination), right
speech, right conduct (behavior), right livelihood, right effort
(suitable striving), right mindfulness (thinking and perception), and right contemplation (absorption) and above all
he laid great stress on right association or company of the holy,
"Truth-winners and arousers of faith" who, through a process
of osmosis (infiltration) instill faith and devotion in the minds
of the aspirants.

Bikkhu Buddharakkita, while describing the *Majjhima Pati-pada,* the Middle Path, or the Golden Mean between the two extremes of self-indulgence and self-mortification, to modern readers, gives us the Buddhistic course of development and discipline through *bhava,* viz.:

1. *Shila Bhavna:* Ethical purity.
2. *Chita Bhavna:* Mental purity.
3. *Pragna Bhavna:* Intuitional insight.

The same author emphasizes the need of developing *shila* or moral purification as the basis of everything else, whether in mundane life or in spiritual advancement. Buddha declared that five benefits accrue to the truly virtuous: good fortune through diligence, fair name abroad, respect in all congregations, clear conscience till the end, and rebirth with a happy destiny.

The basic minimum for the Buddhist layman is the five precepts, or *Panch Shila,* that go to make right conduct or behavior, one of the important steps in the eight-fold path as described above. These are: abstinence from killing, stealing, sexual misconduct, lying, and from drinking intoxicating liquor, and alongside thereof, the observance of positive virtues: *maitri* (friendliness to all), *daan* (charity), *brahmcharya* (chastity), adherence to truth, and temperance. In the Panch Shila of Buddha, we find an exact parallel to the yamas and niyamas as prescribed by the ancients.

The shila, or the process of purification, rests on the two fundamentals: *hiri,* conscience, and *ottappa,* shame; for one rejects evil out of self-respect and scruple on the one hand, and observes respect for another, while the other fears blame or censure. The result is that one develops modesty along with rectitude and propriety. What is true of Buddhism is true also of Jain thought, which enjoins the five great vows of non-violence, non-stealing, non-covetousness, truthfulness and chastity.

This two-fold stress on yamas and niyamas is not just an idiosyncracy of ancient Indian thought. It is to be observed among all people whenever religious experience is actively sought. Thus when we examine the development of Jewish and Christian thought, we come across the same phenomenon. Moses laid down the ten commandments which pointed out the weaknesses to be avoided, namely, worship of gods and deities, engraving images to represent God, vain repetition of God's names, polluting the sabbath, dishonoring one's parents, commission of heinous crimes like killing, adultery and stealing, and lastly, social evils like bearing false witness and coveting a neighbor's house, wife or his belongings (Exodus 20: 4-17). It was left to Jesus to complete the picture when he emphasized the virtues to be developed, in his ten beatitudes: simplicity of spirit, mourning, meekness, hunger and thirst after righteousness, mercy, purity of heart, peace-making, suffering persecution for the sake of righteousness and calmly bearing all manner of reviling and slander (Matthew 5: 1-11). It was not without justice that he claimed, "I have come not to destroy the law but to fulfil the law." The teachings of Islam lay stress on *shariat* (moral injunction), *tauba* (repentance), *faqr* (renunciation), *tazkiya-i-nafs* (subjugation of the senses), *tawakal* (trust in God), *tawhid* (unity) and *zikr* (spiritual discipline), while the Sikh Gurus (prescribing cultivation of essential virtues like chastity, patience, understanding, knowledge, fear of God, austerity, love and compassion), coming much later, reveal a similar pattern. Guru Nanak, in a nutshell, placed true living above everything else:

> *Truth is higher than everything,*
> *But higher still is true living.*
>
> SRI RAG

Why this should be so is not difficult to understand. To be able to progress spiritually, peace and harmony of mind is an absolute necessity. So long as one is the slave of this desire or that, such harmony is impossible. Therefore, one must root out all desires that lead the self away from this harmony. But nature abhors a vacuum; and what is true of physical phenomena is also true of the psychological. The only way to clear the mind of its negative and disintegrating impulses is to replace them by postive and integrating ones. However, while cultivating sadachar, the seeker after truth must remember that it is only a means, not an end, and knowing this, go beyond it to his spiritual goal. Swami Vivekananda, who has analysed the process with great ludicity in *The Secret of Work,* puts the matter thus:

> You must remember that the freedom of the soul is the goal of all yogas . . . A golden chain is as much a chain as an iron one. There is a thorn in my finger, and I use another to take the first out; and when I have taken it out, I throw both of them aside . . . so the bad tendencies are to be counteracted by the good ones, and the bad impressions on the mind should be removed by fresh waves of good ones, until all that is evil disappears, or is subdued. Thus the "attached" becomes the "unattached."

III. Asanas

The term *asana* denotes the seat and the pose, position or posture, in the performance of yogic discipline. It is another external aid in yogic practice. The asana should be steady, firm, pleasant and comfortable, so as to keep the body quiescent but alert during the yogic discipline.

In the Svetasvetara Upanishad II:8 it is said:

> *Keep the upper parts: the chest, the neck, and the head, erect, and subdue within the heart, the senses together with the mind. The wise with the raft of*

Brahman cross over all the powerful torrents of the world.

Similarly, in the Bhagavad Gita VI:11-14 the procedure is laid down as follows:

On a pure spot, he shall set for himself a seat, neither over-high nor over-low, and having over it a cloth, a deer's skin, and kusha grass.

On this couch, he shall seat himself with thought intent and workings of mind and sense instruments restrained, and shall for purification of spirit labor on the Rule.

Firmly, holding the body, head and neck in unmoving equipoise, gazing on the end of his nose and looking not round about him,

Calm of spirit, void of fear, abiding under the vow of chastity, with mind restrained and thought set on me, so shall he sit, who is under the Rule and given over to me.

The term *asana* literally means easy and comfortable. Patanjali enjoined a posture both simple and pleasant (*Yoga Darshana* II:46). That posture is the best which may enable a student of yoga to remain motionless for a long time—two to three hours at a stretch—with an effortless ease, the object being to eliminate bodily reactions and to dissolve the mind into contemplation. Steadiness in asana gives steadiness to the body, and in its turn, to the mind. Theoretically speaking, tradition tells us that there are as many asanas as there are species in the world and as such they run into 8,400,000, but out of these only 84 are important and four are generally accepted as basic and of great value:

(i) *Sukh Asana*: It means easy and comfortable, as it is pleasant to practice. It consists in simply sitting cross-legged, by tucking the left foot under the thigh of the right leg and with open hands resting on the knees, making a circle with the tips of the thumb and the forefinger.

(ii) *Sidh Asana*: This term connotes a disciplined pose, or pose of perfection or attainment. It consists in sitting cross-legged and, in addition to the above, to place the right foot on the left foreleg with heels resting against the pubic bones, without exerting any pressure on the genitals, and palms resting one above the other. It is very useful for attaining *siddhis* or yogic powers and hence the name *sidh asana*. It purifies veins and arteries by supplying fresh blood. It strengthens the heart and lungs, makes breathing deep and slow, regulates the digestive system, and cures diseases like colds, fevers and heart disorders.

(iii) *Padam Asana*: It is a lotus-pose as the name itself implies. In this position, the feet form the petals of a lotus as they cross one over the other. It is rather a difficult pose for persons with stiff joints, but it is very essential for the practice of Hatha Yoga. It is also known as *Anand Asana* for it gives a foretaste of peace and bliss and inclines one to contemplation. It cures the man who practices it of all diseases and ailments, and frees the system from disorders of poisoning and toxins. It rids a person of laziness and languor and mental weakness.

(iv) *Swastika Asana* (the lucky or auspicious pose) : It has all the virtues of its name.

For purposes of spiritual advancement, Sukha or Sidha Asana is admirably suited.

Besides these, some of the well-known asanas are: *Gaoo asana* (the cow pose), *Simha asana* (the lion pose), *Vajra asana* (the thunderbolt pose), *Hal asana* (the plough posture), *Sheersh asana* (the head-stand pose), *Sarvang asana* (the shoulder-stand pose), *Dhanur asana* (the bow pose), *Shava asana* (the corpse pose), *Markat asana* (the monkey pose), *Mayur asana* (the peacock pose), *Kukata asana* (the cock pose), *Garud asana* (the eagle posture), *Ushtr asana* (the camel pose), *Vatyan asana* (the horse pose), *Bhujang asana* (the cobra pose), *Salabh asana* (the locust pose), *Padahast asana, Trikon asana* and *Virksh asana* (the tree pose), etc. This shows the catholicity of the human mind to learn things even from animals and other objects.

Asana as a form of yoga

Some consider asanas as constituting a yoga by themselves and have given them the name of *asana yoga*. But it is not to be used simply for the display of physical feats and skill as some gymnasts do, or as a means of earning a livelihood. It is yoga in the sense that without a disciplined asana, one cannot watch, weed out, and eliminate the *vritis* or the mental currents that keep rising in the mind-stuff or the unfathomable lake of the mind (*chit*). The yoga system is generally divided into two parts: *Pran-kala* or the Path of the Pranas and *Chit-kala* or the Path of the Chit. While Hatha Yoga deals with the Pran-kala, Raja Yoga is concerned with Chit-kala. Asanas form an integral part in both these yogic systems and in fact, are an essential sadhna in every form of yoga whatever it be. Asanas have, on account of their importance, been categorized as a yoga system per se, just as *Dharna* and *Dhyan,* because of their important role in the practice of yoga, have often been described as Dharna Yoga and Dhyan Yoga. The body has of necessity to be set in one posture or position for a considerable time—i.e., three hours—because by continual shifting of posture, one cannot successfully engage in the yogic practice, for with every change of posture the vritis are set in motion and the mind never grows steady and still. Hence the need for a firm and steady pose, but one characterized by ease and comfort, so that the practicer may not feel fatigued and tired during the time he sits for *chit-vriti-nirodha* (elimination of the mental modulations).

Advantages of asanas

Besides being an aid in controlling the mind, the steady asana confers many advantages and these may be classified as follows:

1. Physical advantages:
    (a) The muscular and arterial systems get into proper order.
    (b) The entire body is charged with health, strength and radiant vitality.
    (c) The navel center in the body is fully supplied with heat, which helps in digestion.
    (d) The *pranas,* or the vital airs in the body, begin to function with a regular and rhythmic motion.
    (e) Fearlessness, fortitude and will power come of themselves.
    (f) One gains control over the body and never feels tired, depressed and downcast.
    (g) As one feels inner joy and buoyancy of spirits, his face manifests a healthy radiance.
2. Mental advantages:
    (a) Mind gets steady and well-directed, and one acquires the habit of working with fixed attention.
    (b) Mental freshness.
    (c) Quick understanding and clarity of vision.
    (d) It develops imagination and helps in focusing one's attention or *dhyan.*
    (e) It brings in the habit of deep and concentrated thinking on the otherwise abstruse spiritual problems.
3. Spiritual advantages:
    (a) One, through the recession of physical consciousness due to bodily stability, gradually rises above

the pairs of opposites or state of duality, i.e., hunger and thirst, heat and cold, attachment and detachment, etc.

(b) One easily crosses over the state of *tamogun* (inertia) and *rajogun* (restlessness) and acquires that of *satogun* (peace and equipoise).

(c) One steadily progresses in his sadhna, or spiritual practice, without any fatigue.

Some precautions are generally recommended to secure the sadhak from possible ill effects or obstacles. He should practice the asanas in solitude so that they never become for him a means of exhibiting his virtuosity to the applauding public. It is also advisable that he should avoid proximity to fire, the company of women, undesirable friends, or anything similar that may carry a risk to his body or his mental equilibrium. He must also eschew over-indulgence in food and drink as well as fasting, for the one burdens the body and distracts one's energies, while the other undermines one's vitality. Hence it was that Buddha taught his disciples the middle path, for as he said in his first sermon:

Sensuality is enervating; the self-indulgent man is a slave to his passions, and pleasure-seeking is degrading and vulgar.

And —

by suffering, the emaciated devotee produces confusion and sickly thoughts in his mind. Mortification is not conducive even to worldly knowledge, how much less to a triumph over the senses.

The rule of the golden mean, which applies to everything, applies also to exercise. The understanding sadhak will neither dissipate his energies in over-strenuous exercise like weight-lifting, racing, high or long jumps, nor will he deaden them through lethargy. In short, temperance and simplicity must be the watchwords of his life. Those who specialize in Hatha Yoga or Prana Yoga even go on to lay down the following condition for their day-to-day living:

(a) A place of solitude on a moderate level.
(b) A thatched cottage, preferably square in form, in the midst of natural scenery and verdure.
(c) It should be furnished with a bricked or wooden *takhat* (a raised platfom) to squat upon.
(d) The seat should be covered with palm leaves or dry grass, woollen cover, or a deer-skin.
(e) The site should be so selected as to have a uniformly temperate and even climate all the year round.

All these things should be taken into consideration if one were to choose even a cave (mountain or underground) for spiritual sadhna.

(f) One must exercise scrupulous moderation in his diet and drinks, preferably one helping of porridge in a day.
(g) No outsider should be permitted to haunt the sanctuary.

Gheranda Samhita, a well-known treatise on yoga, gives a detailed account of asanas and the practices allied thereto, viz., *mudras* and *bandhas.* While the mudras are locked postures, the bandhas are fixed postures. The former being psychophysical in nature are generally termed as "gestures," and the latter being purely physical in nature are but "muscular contractions" and are used as catches for holding the pranas at particular places.

While there is quite a large number of mudras, the bandhas are just a few. The well-known mudras or gestures are (1) the *Maha Mudra* (the great gesture), (2) *Maha Bandha,* (3) *Maha Vetha,* (4) *Urgyan (Udlyam),* (5) *Khechari* (moving in the void), (6) *Vajroli,* (7) *Jalandhar,* (8) *Mul-*

vant, (9) *Viprit karna (sauwang),* (10) *Shakti shalana,* or *Prithvi, Ambhavi, Vaishvanari, Vayavi,* and *Akashi* corresponding respectively to the five elements: earth, water, fire, air and ether. In addition to these there are still others like the *Nabho Mudra,* the *Yoni,* the *Manduki,* the *Kaki,* the *Matangi,* the *Bhujangini,* the *Asvini,* etc. Others not enumerated are taken to be modifications of these.

We may make a passing reference to some of them:

(i) *Asvini Mudra:* As the name indicates, it consists in expansion outward and contraction inward of the muscles of the rectum alternately by deep inhalation and exhalation as the *asvini* or mare does after discharging the faeces. It helps in cleansing the intestines, colon and walls, and in expelling the poisonous gases.

(ii) *Vajroli Mudra:* It consists in internal cleanliness of the genitalia by irrigating the general passages in the first instance by oxygenation or air-bath by means of a catheter and then by irrigating them with water mixed with a mild antiseptic. It is performed by *nauli* process, or with the aid of a sprayer or a douche. In its highest technique, one has to withhold the ejaculation of the sex secretions and to re-absorb them into the system.

(iii) *Khechari Mudra* (movement in the void): It consists in retroverting the tongue and pressing it deep into the throat. The practicer gets his tongue split in the form of a fork, as the serpents have. These forked tongues are then washed with a mixed lotion of milk, clarified butter and ashes; and then with the pranic exercise he closes or plugs the two holes of the posterior nostrils by each end of the two-forked tongue and remains absorbed in this condition for days on end and, like a serpent or a tortoise, he may continue in an unconscious state to such an extent that he cannot of himself regain consciousness without the outer aid of others. The whole process is a very complicated one and cannot be practised by a layman with impunity without the aid of a perfect yogin. As the name indicates, the mind remains absorbed in the *khe* or void, as does the tongue in the void of the pharynx.

But this type of samadhi is not a real samadhi with an awakening in cosmic order and a superconscious state, but is a kind of trance in which one altogether loses consciousness itself. This is not the object of true yoga, which aims at *Chaitanya Samadhi* as distinguished from *Jar Samadhi*. A Hatha Yogin through the practice of this mudra can, while drawing his pranas into *Sahasrar,* shut himself in a box, which may be buried underground for months. This kind of Jar Samadhi does not bring in any supersensuous knowledge, wisdom and awareness such as characterizes the fully awakened or Chaitanya Samadhi, which is achieved when the power of consciousness gets established in its own true nature, and which can be terminated at will. That is *Kaivalya* or a state of perfect unison with cosmic and super-cosmic life as contradistinguished from a stone-like, inert state.

For developing concentration, one may practice the following:

(i) *Agochari Mudra* (the imperceptible gesture): Herein one is to sit in his asana with concentration fixed on the nose tip.

(ii) *Bhochari Mudra* (the gesture of the void): Herein the attention is to be fixed on the void, a space four fingers down from the nose-tip up to which the breath flows.

(iii) *Chachari Mudra*: It is called the gesture of the black bee, for in it the mind is to be fixed at the black spot behind the eyes.

While engaged in breath control or *pranayama,* one may practise *Unmani Mudra* or *Kavala Kumbhak.* The latter is a state of dazed intoxication and the other is of peaceful repose.

Again, in the performance of some of the asanas, one has to practice certain muscular contractions or ties, with a view to controlling the vital energy. These contractions or ties are technically called *bandhas*. They are particularly necessary while engaged in pranayama. The most important of these are:

(a) *Mula Bandha* (contraction of the basal plexus) : By it the *Apana Vayu,* or the excretory energy, is locked up and drawn in and upwards to the region of the prana and thus effects, or brings about, a union of the prana with apana, the respiratory with the excretory energies. It is done by pressing the rectum with the heel and a strong inward pull of the breath.

(b) *Jalandhara Bandha:* contraction of the neck plexus where all the arteries meet. It is performed by pressing the chin against the hollow of the collar bones in the chest. It prevents the nectar coming down from Sahasrar from being consumed in the fire within the navel region.

(c) *Uddiyana Bandha:* It consists in contracting the navel muscles so as to give support to the lungs and stomach, during inhalation and exhalation. It also causes the life-breath to flow through the subtle nerve, and hence it also goes by the name of flying contraction.

Perfection in asanas (Asana Siddhi)

There are three signs of perfection in *Asana Siddhi* :

1. During the time of asana, the body should be in a state of perfect repose and relaxation, with no movement in any part thereof.

2. Again, one should rise above body-consciousness, and have no knowledge even of sensory and motor currents, which are to be left to themselves with no thought about them.

3. Last, but not the least, one should feel and actually enjoy happiness and bliss within him.

One can acquire Asana Siddhi or discipline in a year by practicing it regularly for one to six hours every day.

However, before proceeding further in our survey of Patan-jali's Ashtang Yoga, we must remind ourselves that a mastery of the asanas and temperance in living are to be looked upon as a means and not as the end. The sadhak must not forget that physical culture is a preparation. Just as he used ethics with its yamas and niyamas to purify his mind for the inner journey, so too he must discipline his body and daily living, and then work toward his ultimate goal: at-one-ment with Brahman. This point needs emphasizing because human nature is such that in pursuing an arduous course, it often forgets the final end, setting up the means as the goal. Many a yogin takes to the development of physical culture as though that were the be-all and end-all of yoga. In such cases, success in practice of asanas and in moderation of needs, instead of preparing the way for further progress, brings with it a sense of pride and vanity resulting in complacency and spiritual inertia. The discriminating sadhak will learn the basic essentials from this branch of yoga—the secret of health and the best posture for meditation—but he will not attempt to specialize in it or to master all its refinements, for he will know that to get absorbed in the means is to forget the end.

Food

"As is the food, so is the mind," is an ancient saying, and in it lies an incontrovertible truth, for it is food that goes to make the body and the brain.

Satvic food plays an important part in the perfection of the body as envisaged by Hatha Yoga, and helps in carrying on any sadhna or yogic discipline without fatigue, languor, lassitude or drowsiness. The chart on the opposite page lists some of the foods which help or retard the yogic sadhna.

In brief, fresh and green vegetables, leafy vegetables, fruits and nuts, milk, butter and ghee constitute an ideal diet for any man. Three meals a day are considered more than suffi-

Hatha Yoga Foods

Foods conducive to the yogic sadhna	Foods that retard the yogic sadhna
1 Barley, black gram, whole mung (green gram), rice, til (gingelly seeds), shakar (jaggery), milk and milk products, butter and clarified butter — all in moderation.	Moth, mash, musur (lentils), peas, unhusked gram, wheat, oils and fats, sour milk and sour curd, spoiled ghee, meat in all forms, fish, fowl and eggs, etc.
2 Black pepper, almonds, ginger, currants, lime— in moderation.	Pineapple, red radishes.
3 Mangoes, grapes, guavas, apples, oranges, figs, gooseberries, dates and peaches, etc. — in moderation.	Watermelon and kakari.
4 Melon, cucumber — in small quantities.	Turi (snake gourd), kashiphal (red pumpkin), brinjal (eggplant), lady's finger and chulai (amaranth or spinach-like plant).
5 Pumpkin, plain turi (ridge gourd), ghia turi (plain gourd), spinach, parwal (coecinia indica) and swaran leaves — in small quantities.	Spices, condiments, chilies, pepper, sauces and other acid producing stimulants and things pungent, bitter and sour.

cient. We may note that foods that are stale, highly seasoned, half-cooked or over-cooked, and fruits that are over-ripe or under-ripe or lying cut; also sweets and sweetmeats, are to be avoided. Likewise, aerated drinks, stimulants like tea and coffee, and intoxicants of all descriptions are not to be brought into use.

IV. PRANAYAM OR YOGIC BREATHING

He who knows prana, knows the Vedas.

SANTIS

Before dealing with *pranayam,* it is necessary to know what the *pranas* (the vital airs) are, their classification and functions, etc., in the body and how they act and the things allied with them. Prana is the sum total of all energy that is manifest in the Universe, the sum total of all the forces in Nature. Heat, light, electricity, magnetism, gravitation, etc., are all manifestations of prana. All forces, all powers and even the pranas themselves spring from one and the same source—the fountainhead of atman. *Pran tatwa* is much superior to *manas tatwa* or the mind-principle, of which Nanak says:

He who conquers the mind, conquers the world.

The motor power behind the mind-stuff, as said already, is that of prana and hence the regulation and control of prana, the primal force in the Universe, is of prime importance and far above other psycho-physical disciplines. In the *Gorakh Samhita* it is said that he who knows the secret of prana knows the secret of yoga, for in the rhythmic regulation of prana lies the practical aspect of yoga par excellence.

Pranas are classified into five important categories according to the nature of their functions:

(a) *Prana* is concerned with the respiratory system. It is the breath of life and, like a bird in a cage, gives vitality to the human system. Its seat is said to be in the region lying between the two eyebrows, called *chid-akash,* up to which place the field of its operation extends.

(b) *Apana* helps the excretory system, as it has a tendency to flow downwards. It operates in the region below the navel.

(c) *Samana* aids the digestive organs. It is so called as it conducts equally the food to the entire system. Its seat is in the navel and it spreads on all sides, nourishing the body as a whole.

(d) *Udana* is connected with deglutition; it is named from its quality of ascending, drawing or guiding breath. Its movement is perceptible between the navel and the head. Its seat is in the neck and it has a tendency to fly upwards.

(e) *Vyana* helps in maintaining the circulatory system in the entire body. It affects internal division and diffusion and is so called from its pervading (*vyapati*) the body like the ethereal element.

Besides these primary pranas, there are five other kinds of lesser importance, namely:

(i)   *Naga* which helps belching or eructation.
(ii) *Kurma* is connected with the eyes, and helps the blinking process and induces sleep.
(iii) *Krikala* pervades through the facial muscles and spreads out in the act of sneezing.
(iv) *Deva-datta* brings about yawning and takes one into a gentle sleep.
(v)   *Dhanan-jay* is associated with the work of assimilation.

These vital airs pervade the skin, bones, muscles, tendons, ligaments and the like.

Plexuses and chakras

Wherever several nerves, arteries or veins interlace each other, that point or center is called a plexus. Similarly, there are plexuses or centers of vital forces in the *Suksham* or subtle *nadis* and these are called *chakras* or *padmas*. The *nadis* are the astral tubes made up of astral matter, and serve as passages for subtle pranas through which they operate in the subtle body as do the nerves, arteries and veins in the gross physical body. All these subtle tubes or nadis spring from *Kanda* or the center where the *Sushmana Nadi* meets the *Muladhana Chakra* at the base of the spine. Of these nadis, *Ida, Pingala* and *Sushmana* are the most important. All three nadis are within the spinal cord. Ida and Pingala are on the left and right side respectively of the Sushmana or Sukhman. The Ida (*Chandra* canal) flows through the right. Breath generally flows through each for about two hours alternately. But when it flows through the Sushmana (*Agni* canal), the mind becomes steady. This steadiness or *Unmani Avastha,* as it is called, is the highest state in Raja Yoga, for in this state there is wonderful meditation. The practice of Pranayam is necessary for purification of the nadis, as with impurities in them, the breath cannot pass through the middle nadi.

Gross prana travels in the nerves of the physical body, but the subtle prana moves in the astral tubes (nadis). The breath is an external effect of the manifestation of the gross prana.

There is a very close and intimate connection between the gross and the subtle prana. If the mind and the prana cease to vibrate, no thought-waves will arise.

> *The mind functions through prana,*
> *It is from prana (life) that everything proceeds.*
> CHHANDOGYA UPANISHAD

When prana departs from the body, all organs cease to function, for in the body there is no greater force than bionergy (prana).

Pranayam: Elementary exercises

Hatha Yoga Pradipka lays great stress on yogic breathing for "all life exists only from breath to breath," and it said that "he who breathes half, only lives half." We must therefore develop air-hunger. For "vital airs," says Hippocrates, "is the real *pabulum vitae.*" Deep breathing is a great, positive aid to self-culture and helps in retaining health, youth and longevity. The habit of conscious deep breathing gives a good exercise to the respiratory organs and ensures a free circulation of blood. Respiration consists of alternate expansion and contraction as the air is drawn in or expelled out from the lungs, and these are termed inhalation (inspiration) and exhalation (expiration) respectively. Each of these is followed by a suspensory pause within and without. Thus pranayam has four processes, namely: *Puraka* or inhalation, *Antar Kumbhak* or retention within, and *Rechaka* or exhalation followed by *Vahya Kumbhak* or *Sunyaka,* i.e., expiratory pause. This can be done through both the nostrils very, very slowly, and should be repeated ten to twenty times in the morning and in the evening for about three months. One may start with Puraka and Rechaka and after some time add the other two practices of standstill pauses (Antar and Vahya Kumbhaka) for a few seconds. By practice and perseverance, one can acquire efficiency in yogic breathing. The suspending of breath at will after in-breathing or out-breathing, is called *Kevalya Kumbhaka.*

Sukh Purvak Pranayam
(Easy and comfortable form of pranayam)

Sitting on Padam or Sukh Asana, one should close the right nostril with the thumb of the right hand and exhale the air slowly and rhythmically in one long and unbroken expiration through the left nostril. Now the left nostril is also to be closed with the little or ring finger of the right hand and the Vahya Kumbhak be maintained as long as possible without the least discomfort. Then the breath is to be inhaled, very, very, slowly, through the right nostril after removing the thumb which is to be followed by Antar Kumbhak. Then the order is to be reversed. All these eight processes constitute one pranayam. One ought to commence with five to ten pranayams in the morning and in the evening, on an empty stomach, and gradually increase the same to twenty, together with increased Kumbhak or retention without causing any inconvenience. While doing pranayam, one should think that *Divya Sampardie* (Niyamas) like mercy, compassion, love, peace and joy, are being absorbed in the system and *Asuraya Sampardie* (Yamas) like anger, lust, greed and selfishness, are being discarded and ejected by the system. It would be well to do *Simran,* if one may like, during the pranayam.

In the higher stages of Pranayam, the vital breath rises in the Sushmana Nadi and flows toward *Sahasrar.* The movement is felt in the first instance like that of an ant, and gradually grows into that of a frog, till with the clearing and purification of the nadi through continued practice, the prana begins to fly like a bird.

There are different types of breath-controlling processes, e.g.:

(i) Out-breathing and in-breathing through both nasal channels combined with Kumbhaka.

(ii) Out-breathing and in-breathing through one of the nasal channels at a time followed by Kumbhaka. It is called *Surya Bhedana* and *Chandra Bhedana,* when performed through the right and left sides respectively.

(iii) In-breathing through both and out-breathing though one of the nasal passages at a time.

(iv) *Shitkari* and *Shitali*: These are two forms of sipping and sucking the air through pouted lips, along the tongue (after closing both the nostrils), and after holding the air a little deep down, to release it through the nostrils. This is just like drinking the vital breath through the crow-beak.

(v) *Bhasrika*: It consists in taking breaths in quick succession through one channel at a time, and then slowly exhaling the last breath through the other channel and vice versa. It is just like working the bellows and hence is called bellows-breathing or *Bhasrika*.

Pranayam, or yogic breathing, can be practiced profitably and successfully under the guidance of a Guru or an adept in the method and by those who observe truthfulness, continence, temperance, moderation in diet, humility and patience, are not given to any kind of addictions, and above all, are free from heart and lung diseases and congenital disorders.

The great achievement of pranayam is to awaken and bring into full play the coiled serpentine energy of Kundalini, lying in a dormant state at the spinal root-center. As it rises higher and higher in the Sukhman, the various subtle centers in the subtle nadis get illuminated, till it reaches Sahasrar, the fountain of light. With the destruction of the veil over the Radiance of Eternity, the mind gets quickly absorbed and concentration follows of itself.

The muscular and nerve control by the practice of asanas is but a preparatory stage, and the real technique of yoga begins with the harnessing of the vital pranas or the ten engines in the body.

Pranayam brings *Chit Shudhi, Manas Shudhi* and *Nadi Shudhi* and thereby steadies the mind and helps in concentration, and in destroying the coverings or koshas on the soul. It removes all desires, improves designation and helps in maintaining *brahmcharya* (continence) and attaining *ekagrata* (one-pointedness) and *kumbhaka* (state of peace), with or without *purak* or *rechaka,* or the inhaling and exhaling processes.

Pranayam should be done after answering the call of nature and after thorough cleansing of the nares or nasal channels with pure and tepid water, and by gargling the throat.

It should be practised all alone in a sitting posture in a room with open windows to let in fresh air and with the mouth closed. After fifteen minutes of the practice, a cup of milk does good. Bathing is to be avoided immediately after such exercises.

The object of pranayam is to restrain the vritis of the mind and to make the mind-stuff steady, like the jet of a lamp in a windless place. All *abhyas* or practice whatsoever is directed to driving the mind to its source—*Hirdey Guha*—and to get it absorbed in atman.

The evil vritis of the mind can be removed by cultivating good vritis, so as to replace lust (*kam*) by continence (*brahmcharya*), pride (*madha*) by humility (*nimrta*), greed (*lobh*) by contentment (*santosh*), niggardliness by magnanimity, delusion by discrimination, dishonesty by honesty, fickleness by determination, arrogance by politeness, jealousy by nobility, attachment by detachment, enmity by friendliness, and so on.

The Vedantic method consists in cutting the branches of *sankalpa* from the tree of the mind (*manas*), and then destroying the tree itself by cutting the roots in the ego.

Pranayam as a form of yoga
(The Prana Yoga)

The importance of pranayam as an integral part of Hatha Yoga and Raja Yoga is so great, that some have come to regard it as an independent form of yoga in itself and have given it the name of Prana Yoga.

As explained already, the Ida and Pingala nadis starting from *svadhistan chakra,* the center of life-breath, run spirally round the central nadi, Sukhmana, and end in the left and right nostril respectively. Ida is influenced by the moon, while Pingala is influenced by the sun. Ida has in abundance the moisture of the moon and represents the female principle, while Pingala has the energy of the sun and represents the male principle in nature. Both of these nadis, the negative and the positive, work under the action of *prakriti* and *purush,* i.e., matter and soul combined.

When the Pingala Nadi, which is influenced by the energy of the sun, is in active motion, the food taken is easily and quickly digested. When the Ida Nadi starts, it brings in strength and vitality to the system and helps in the development of the body and bodily muscles, etc. It is under the active influence of both these heavenly bodies, as operating through these nadis, that further growth takes place both in nature and in the human species, both female and male. The moisture of the moon helps the production of *raj* in women, and the life-giving energy of the sun that of *viraj* or semen in men.

During the daytime, the solar nadi (Pingala) operates for most of the time, and hence the food should be taken while the live energy of the sun is in active motion so it will get easily dissolved in the system and thus become the source of strength. Food taken at night after the setting of the sun is likely to increase body bulk and fats and to create digestive disorders, which may lead to disturbance in the equilibrium of the elemental constituents in the body, like *kaf* (phlegm), *safra* (heat) and *sauda* (gaseous vibrations), etc.

Pranic discipline

This discipline, in brief, consists in setting up:

(a) Some center within the body, say at the plexus of the heart or the region of the vital airs, where the *mano-mai-atman* dwells.

(b) Some center outside the body.

(c) One has to work at both the centers within and without and to do pranayam in between the two centers.

(d) The practice of *tratak* or the discipline of the vision (sight), by gradually bringing the attention from without to within, and keeping it fixed on one of these inner centers for some time.

In setting up centers outside the body one has to sit in solitude and make a yellow spot on a white paper, which is to be placed on the table or hung on the wall on a level with the eyes. *Tratak* or the fixing of the gaze is then done on that spot while the pingala nadi is in action. The attention is also to be fixed on and gradually absorbed within the *Anahat* Sound. After practicing this for a few days, the outer spot is to be changed to blue, to red, to bluish white, and lastly into a brilliantly white color, after some days of practice at each colored spot. The object of the tratak practice (spot-gazing) is to have a clear vision of the elemental colors which are representative of the colors of earth, water, fire, air and ether, respectively. For quicker results, this is to be done for at least two or three hours every day. It improves eyesight and serves as a great aid in influencing others.

Again, one has to take care of the distance between the spot and the organ of sight. To begin with, the spot is to be located at a distance of about two feet; after practicing for a few days, the distance is to be reduced to one and three-fourths feet, to one foot and then to half a foot. When this tratak develops ino a kind of exhilarating absorption, it may be brought still nearer to the tip of the nose. Then begins the real sadhna and gradually the attention is to be brought to the root of the nose between the two eyebrows. The importance of this practice is that the scattered vritis are to be controlled from wandering without, collected at the still-point in the body or the seat of the mind, and inverted within to bring them in contact with the Anahat Sound. This also brings about, of itself, rhythm in the pranas, and both the vritis and the pranas simultaneously get adjusted of themselves. By the process of tratak, the mind and the pranas become harmonized, and the soul escapes through the mano-mai and pran-mai koshas, or the covering sheaths.

Advantages of Prana Yoga

The practice of Prana Yoga helps in developing all the sense faculties, viz., perception, audition, olfaction, touch and taste. A yogin can, by his thought-force, attract to his aid from the atmosphere all the powers that he may like, by relating them to his thought. In bitter cold winter, a sadhak may sit in sidh asana with his chin fixed on his chest, think of the sun, and start the practice with pingala or the solar nadi. Heat would generate of itself and cover him with perspiration. In the same way one can, in the mid-summer heat, have the experience of cold. All this depends on thought-force, provided one knows how to fix his attention at the seat of the soul. This is the height of Prana Yoga. One can develop all these powers by bringing the mind and the pranas to one common level. Thought-force springs from the mind, and Prana Yoga consists in bringing the prana into unison with the mind at the level of the soul, or the divine plane.

V. Pratyahara or Sense Control
(Withdrawal and Abstraction)

This means withdrawal of the senses from the sense-objects. The mind is rendered pure by the practice of yamas, niyamas and pranayama, while *pratyahara* gives supreme mastery over the senses. The control of the senses, therefore, is the primal factor in the yogic science. Unless the sense steeds are controlled and checked in their mad career in the fields of enjoyment and pleasure, the mind cannot possibly be stilled. The senses have, therefore, to be withdrawn from the sensory plane and protected from taking in all outer impressions and influences. Visual perception and audition are the two main inlets from which we derive no less than 88 to 95 per cent of our impressions, and the remaining five per cent or so come from the other senses. Thus, it is of paramount importance to close down the sluice-gates of the eyes and ears to prevent the outer floodwaters from entering and inundating the lake of the mind. To shut the mind resolutely against the onslaughts of the senses, it is necessary for the student of yoga to retire for some time every day into the "monastic cell" of his heart, for it is a matter of common experience that muddy water becomes clear of itself if it is allowed to stand for some time.

One can practice pratyahara (control of senses as a preliminary to attaining a state of reverie or sensory withdrawal) through discrimination and discernment. With the knowledge of the true values of life, we come to disregard the unhealthy and unworthy food in which otherwise the senses indulge, and thereby come to control the mindstuff. It is tantamount to dislocating the sense traffic in the world by dynamiting the fields of illusory pleasures with the power of discrimination. Pratyahara is very essential for achieving success in yoga. With the senses inverted, a yogin can work for the consciousness within him. By its practice, the mind becomes purified, grows strong in self-reliance, and is enabled to lead a strictly austere life.

In the Bhagavad Gita, we have:

> Let him hold all these (senses) in constraint and concentrate upon me; for he who has his sense instruments under his sway has wisdom abidingly set.

The above five factors—*yamas, niyamas, asanas, pranayam* and *pratyahara*—constitute a preparation for progress in yoga. They are but accessories to, and not the main elements of, the yogic system. They help in purifying the body, the pranas, the mind and the indriyas.

Now we come to the direct internal aids to yoga. These are

three in number, viz., *dharna, dhyan* and *samadhi,* which constitute *Antarang Sadhna* or inner discipline.

VI. DHARNA OR SAMYAM
(ABSORPTION OR CONCENTRATION)

Having controlled the pranas through pranayam, and the senses through pratyahara, the student of yoga has now to fix his mind on something. It may be fixed on something without, like an idol or a picture, or any other kind of representation; or it may be fixed on something within, on any of the bodily centers in the *pind,* or on any idea or on any of the astral centers in the *und.* Dharna, then, consists in fixing the mind on a particular place, object, idea or center, as one may find convenient. Any type of dharna helps in making the mind steady and is beneficial in its own way.

(i) Dharna on any of the sense perceptions provides steadiness to the mind by collecting the wandering wits at the focal point.

(a) On the tip of the nose, it gives an experience of *divya gandh* or divine fragrance. It is called *varta siddhi.*

(b) On the tip of the tongue, it gives the experience of the taste of divya essence or divine-stuff; manna and nectar. The divine knowledge of taste is known as *asvadan.*

(c) On the middle of the tongue, it gives the experience of the divya touch or proximity of the sublime presence. The divine knowledge of touch is known as *vidana.*

(d) On the root of the tongue, it gives the experience of divya sounds or holy harmony. It is called *sravana.*

(e) On the palate or roof over the tongue, it gives the experience of the divya colors or elemental brilliance. This divine knowledge of sight is called *adarsha*.

(ii) Dharna on the luminous mental state at the seat of the mind: It is practised first by inhaling and then exhaling the breath, together with the thought of turning into an upward position the eight-petaled lotus below the heart, lying at present face downwards, and then fixing the attention on the effulgent light in the lotus through which passes the Sushmana or the Brahm Nadi.

(iii) Dharna on Master-souls like Buddha, Christ or prefereably still, a living Master, who are freed from all desires also frees one from all desires, mental attachments and the bondage of mind and matter.

(iv) Dharna or samyam on external objects: Dharna on heavenly bodies like the sun, the moon, the planets, etc., gives supersentient experience, e.g.:

(a) On the sun it gives the knowledge of the Brahmand consisting of fourteen bhavans or regions; seven upper or higher worlds or *lokas* (*bhur, bhuva, swah, maha, janah, tapah* and *satyam*), and seven lower or nether lokas (*sutala, vitala talatala, mahatala, rasatala, atala* and *patala*).

(b) On the moon, it gives the knowledge of the stars.

(c) On the pole-star, it gives the knowledge of the movement of the stars.

(d) On the elephant or *hanuman*, it gives strength and valor.

(e) On the form of the body, it causes disappearance of the body itself, as the power of comprehension is checked and the connection between the light and the eyes is severed.

(v) Samyam on internal centers, the self, and indriyas: Dharna or samyam may be practiced on anything like virtues, internal centers, chakras and nadis, as for example:

(a) On the *nabhi* or navel (*manipura chakra*), it gives the knowledge of the construction of the body.

(b) On the pit of the throat (*vishudhi chakra*), it gives freedom from hunger and thirst.

(c) On the *Sahasrar,* it gives divine visions and *darshan* of the *siddhas.*

The method of the last is by concentrating on *Brahmarendra* or the whole of Brahma, which is an aperture within the *mundhu* or head through which divine light flows downwards. *Nirgun upasakas* carry on their abstract meditation on this center, which is also known as *Sahasrar.*

(d) On the *anhat chakra* at the heart, it gives the knowledge of the mind.

(e) On *kurma nadi* (the astral tube in the chest, below the throat, and through which *kurma* or the sub-prana works the eyelids), it gives steadiness to the body.

(f) On the inner light of the heart, it gives the knowledge of the subtle (clairvoyance), the obscure (buried treasures), the remote (far and wide).

(vi) One may do samyam on one's own self. It gives clairvoyance, clairaudience, and other transcendental powers, also higher touch, higher taste and higher smell, etc., all through intuition or *pratibha,* without any of the other specialized samyams.

By samyam on one's own essential nature (the cognitive powers), one gets the power of pure cognition without the outer aids of the senses and the sense-organs. With the indriyas lying dormant in their respective centers, one enjoys ineffable bliss (*anand*) in a state called *Sanand Samadhi.*

(vii) By samyam or dharna on certain features of the body, such as the complexion, the voice, or any other thing, one begins to understand the state and the nature of the minds of others.

(viii) By samyam:

(a) On mind (or mental thoughts), one knows the contents of the mind.

(b) On time, one gets knowledge of everything.

(c) On air and ether or on the relation between the two, one is endowed with the divine hearing (*shabd*), and can hear any subtle sound from any distance simply by his will. Similarly, by contacting the *adhistana-bhutas* (*vayu tejas* and *prithvi, etc.*), one can develop powers of other organs to their fullest capacity.

(d) On the relation between ether and body, or on the lightness of cotton, comes the power of flying through ether or air, for the body becomes extremely light, and one can move anywhere in space like a bird and can even ride on the rays of the sun.

A yogin having *siddhi* in *Kechari Mudra* can also fly in the air. (One who knows *Sammohan Vidya* or *Indra Jala* can also move through space, but this is *jala* or a trick only, and not something real, for he actually remains on the ground and if you were to photograph him, you will not get the photo of such a man flying through the air.)

(e) On the three modifications of mind, comes the knowledge of the past and future.

(f) On *videha,* one can pass out of the body at will and function without the body, feel the all-pervading nature in its full omnipresence and can perform *kaya parvesh,* i.e., can enter into the body of any other human being and operate through his body and mind.

(g) On *samskaras* (impressions of mind), comes the knowledge of previous births.

(ix) By mastery over:

(a) *Udana vayu,* one ceases to have any contact with water, mud or thorns, and can end his existence at will, for through *udana,* one can separate his astral body from the physical body and travel through space.

(b) *Samana vayu,* comes effulgence and one can create fire and flashes of light from one's body.

(x) By samyam on virtues:

(a) On friendliness and other virtues, comes the power to transmit the same to others.

(b) On discrimination (on the distinctive relation between *satva* or purity and *purusha* or the soul), comes the power of omnipotence and omniscience.

(c) On *shabda,* comes the knowledge of the sounds of all living beings (including those of animals and birds).

(d) On the karmas, one gets the knowledge of the time of his death.

When the mind becomes extremely pure and is filled with *satva* through and through to its very roots, spontaneous illumination dawns. The mind has five states:

(a) *Kshipta,* or the wandering mind, with mind-stuff in a state of continued dispersion.

(b) *Mudha,* or the mind that is dull and forgetful and knows next to nothing. In it, the mind is in a state of confusion and stupidity.

(c) *Vikshipta,* or the mind that collects and gathers in momentarily and then fritters away. It is a state of imperfect stability.

(d) *Ekagrata,* or the mind gifted with one-pointed attention and fixity of purpose.

(e) *Nirodha,* or the mind that is disciplined, controlled and well-restrained.

No yoga is possible in the first three states. It is possible only in the fourth and fifth states.

In addition to the above, there are eight kinds of *siddhis,* or powers, which siddhas or the superior beings generally exercise:

(a) *Anima* — capacity to penetrate into all things, even an *anu* or atom, so as to see into its inner structure.

(b) *Laghima* — capacity to acquire lightness, so as to ride even on the rays of the sun. It is often made use of in levitation and translevitation, in spite of the laws of gravitation.

(c) *Garima* — capacity to become as heavy as steel and to make any object immovable. It is the opposite of *laghima.*

(d) *Mahima* — capacity to acquire extensive and all-pervading magnitude like space, and to see the working of universal order and far-off things like solar systems.

(e) *Prapti* — capacity to reach anywhere, even to the moon. It endows one with a sense of all pervasiveness.

(f) *Prakamyam* — capacity to have all desires fulfilled.

(g) *Vasitvam* — capacity to command and control all creatures and elemental forces, like the wind and the rain, etc.

(h) *Ishitva* — capacity to play the creator, the preserver and the destroyer.

Besides these, there are many subsidiary attainments which

one gets by the simple process of self-control and concentration, also called samyams, e.g.:

    (i) To understand the language of birds and beasts.

   (ii) To know one's previous births and to have foreknowledge of death.

  (iii) To read the innermost thoughts of others.

  (iv) To know of secret and subtle things from afar, like the planets and the stars.

   (v) To foretell future events.

  (vi) To transport oneself to any place in the world.

 (vii) To heal by touch.

(viii) To gain bodily perfections in *rupa* (form), *ranga* (complexion), *bala* (strength and fortitude), *sanhanan* (steadiness) and *lavanya* (physical charm), etc.

It is necessary here to give a word of caution regarding riddhis and siddhis, or the supernatural powers that one very often comes to acquire in the practice of yoga sadhna or yogic discipline. They are to be scrupulously avoided, as they are positive obstacles in the way of true spiritual progress and the attainment of self-realization and God-realization, which are the aim and end of the yoga system. The *devtas* very often get jealous of the human soul travelling on the Spiritual Path. They come to greet with smiles the yogins who find an ingress into higher regions, invite them with sweet and cunning words, and try to bring about their downfall. Even the great yogin Vishvamitra was allured by the beauty of a celestial being, a maiden, sent by Indra to tempt him. He unwittingly fell into the snare and fell from the Path. These temptations assail one in the second stage of the journey, but prove of no avail to one who adheres to the Path, and is firm and steadfast in his sadhna.

Give up siddhis and destroy the seeds of bondage,

> *And attain Kevalya, the state of perfect ease and*
> *independence.*

Again:

> *Be not allured by the winning smiles of the celestials,*
> *And avoid contact with all that is undesirable.*

PATANJALI

Dharna as a form of yoga (Mansik Yoga)

Fixity of attention is the essential primary element in the internal yoga sadhna, and its importance cannot be overrated. "When the senses are stilled, the mind is at rest, and the intellect wavers not—that, say the wise, is the highest state." (Katha Upanishad II: iii-10). It is because of the fact that it occupies a pivotal position in the system, that it is regarded by some as a form of yoga by itself, and they give it the name of *Mansik* or mental yoga (the yoga of self-absorption).

Most of the students devote themselves wholly and solely to the strict observance of yamas and niyamas only, and as such hardly make any headway on the Path of yoga proper, which aims at self-realization and God-realization. Those who do go ahead a little, do not get further than yogic postures (asanas, mudras, and bandhas), and are preoccupied with body building processes and muscular development, making them the sole aim of all their endeavors. They confine themselves to the physical culture aspect of yoga, so as to defy disease, senility and an early death. A few fortunate souls who progress to pranayam make it the be-all and the end-all of the yogic sadhna and, taking pleasure in contracting their pranas in the *Brahmarendra,* spend most of their time like a tortoise in their shell in *yoga nidra,* regarding inertness as the highest form of samadhi. All of these are but means to the higher purposes of yoga and should only be practiced as such. The goal of yoga is self-realization by a regular process of self-analysis and withdrawal, so as to enable one to rise above body-consciousness into higher cosmic and super-cosmic consciousness.

True yoga is a natural process with no artifice in it. It should be readily intelligible and easy to practice. But for lack of proper teachers, well-versed in the theory and practice of yoga, it has become a burdensome thing and an intricate affair, too difficult to understand and still more difficult to practice. Today, life has grown too complex to allow any man the leisure and the opportunity to master all the branches of yoga (each of which has grown more specialized with the passage of time), and then to proceed to the final goal. The result is that aspirants begin to mistake this or that branch of yoga as the ultimate, and fritter away their energy in its pursuit, content merely with the acquisition of physical or magical powers.

In actual experience, the mind in a state of *sushupti* (or deep slumber) does come to coincide in some measure with the lower blissful plane (*anand*) and the lower cognitive plane (*vigyan*), for on waking up, one carries with him into consciousness the impression of the undisturbed and unalloyed bliss enjoyed in the deep sleep. But this is an involuntary experience in the *pind* or the sensory plane and not one consciously acquired at will. With a proper understanding and practice of the real sadhna, one can boldly lift the veil and have a dip in the fount of bliss on a spiritual level, whenever he may like, and may remain internally in contact with the life-current itself, which is the very source of true bliss and happiness. Just as by pranayam, one can contact the pranas with the mind, so in the same way by pratyahara and dharna, one can contact the mind-plane with the plane of cognition in the higher spiritual centers above.

The term *pratyahara* means "restraint," and hence it denotes restraining the mindstuff and the senses from flowing out into the world and running about in search of sense pleasures from sense objects. But this is hardly possible unless the senses and the mind are provided with something akin to, or more pleasing than, the worldly objects, which may serve as an anchor to keep the senses and mind fixed within. This is called *dharna,* which means "to accept" and "to be absorbed" in the object of concentration. Pratyahara and dharna go together; for on the one hand the mind is to be weaned away from the worldly pleasures without, and on the other hand, is to be provided with something more attractive within.

The yogins, while sitting in some asana, first control the navel plexus and then drawing the pranas to the heart plexus, bring them to coincide with the mind-plane, after which, by various practices like tratak on some higher center, they try to invert the mind and make it recede. The first part is called pratyahara and the second, of recession and absorption in the higher center, is called dharna.

The mind, by sheer force of habit extending over ages upon ages, has acquired a tendency to run after pleasures. The pleasures of the world may be categorized into five classes as follows:

(a) *Rup* and *rang,* or beautiful forms, designs, and colors which may attract the eye.

(b) *Shabd* or melodies, tuneful and enchanting, as may capture the ear.

(c) *Ras* or delectable victuals and viands as may captivate the palate.

(d) *Gandh* or fragrant scents as may directly appeal to the olfactory sense.

(e) *Sparsh* or physically pleasing sensations as come from touch.

In a waking state with the senses alert, one enjoys the physical aspects of the pleasures as enumerated above. In a dream state, which is more or less a reflex of the astral or subtle, one enjoys sound the most, for in that state it has a direct appeal to the mind. In the dreamless and deep sleep state, which is a reflex of the causal or seed state, one gets cognition of deep absorption.

One has, therefore, to draw himself within to the heart center by means of tratak on different elemental colors connected with ether, air, fire, water and earth, and they will grow into enchanting refulgence. By regular practice, the yogins acquire supernatural powers and capacities to taste all the five pleasures mentioned above in their subtle form from a far distance. These powers come naturally with the coincidence of pranas with the mind.

The practice of pratyahara and dharna can be still further developed with the help of tratak, until one can move and recede inwards and upwards from the heart center to the thyroid or throat center (*kanth chakra*) and thereby contact the cognitive plane. This movement from a lower center to a higher one results from the practice both of pratyahara, which enables one to leave the center below, and of dharna, whereby one takes hold of and gets absorbed in the next higher center. This process continues until one reaches *aggya chakra,* which is located behind and between the two eyebrows, the headquarters of the soul as it functions in the physical world in the waking state.

As the sensory currents collect together and gather at this center, and one, forgetting about himself, rises above body-consciousness, there dawns in him by degrees, the inner spiritual light, which with great absorption or dharna grows into greater effulgence. With perfection in dharna or complete absorption at this stage, all the centers down to the *mul* or *guda* chakra at the rectum, become illumined.

In this connection, we may here refer to the physiology of the yoga system. The cerebro-spinal system is the mainstay of the body. The spinal column in yogic terminology is called

Meru or *Brahm Danda.* According to the *Shiva Samhita,* there are in the human system as many as 350,000 nadis, and out of these, the following ten play an important part:

(i) *Ida*: Starting from the lowest plexus (*guda chakra*), on the right side of the spinal column, it extends spirally around the sushmana and goes as far as the left nostril.

(ii) *Pingala*: Starting from the same chakra on the left side of the spinal column, it extends spirally as far as the right nostril.

(iii) *Sushmana* or *Sukhmana*: Is the central nadi in between the ida and pingala nadis and runs through the spinal column from the guda chakra to the Great Aperture, known as *Brahmarendra,* behind and between the eyebrows.

(iv) *Gandhari*: Comes to the left eye, after rising from the front of the central nadi.

(v) *Hastijivha*: Comes to the right eye, after rising from the rear of the central nadi.

(vi) *Pushpa*: Comes to the right ear from the central nadi.

(vii) *Yashvini*: Comes to the left ear from the central nadi.

(viii) *Alambhush*: Stretches to the root of the arms.

(ix) *Kuhu* or *Shubha*: It goes down to the tip of the generative organ.

(x) *Shankhni*: It goes down to the rectum.

The first three, the ida, pingala and sushmana nadis, are the most important. The ida and pingala nadis, before entering into the base of the nostrils, cross each other and are known as gangliated cords.

The third one, the sushmana or sukhmana, or the central nadi, passes through the spinal column and runs through six plexuses or centers as follows:

(a) *Muladhara* (Basal Plexus) with a four-petaled lotus, extending on four sides.

Chart of the Chakras or Plexuses

No.	Seat of the Ganglionic Centers	Presiding Deities (Hindu and Sufi)	Associated Elements	Representative Colors	Functions of Each Center	Merits of Meditation Thereon
1	Guda (rectum)	Ganesh	Earth	Yellow	Purification of the body	It rids one of all ailments and grants the capacity to fly in the air (levitation)
2	Indri (generative organ)	Brahma (Michael)	Water	Blue	Creation of species	Fearlessness, freedom from all bondage
3	Nabhi (navel)	Vishnu (Israel)	Fire	Red	Sustenance and preservation of species	Lord of all desires; heals all diseases; seer of hidden treasures; ability to enter into other bodies
4	Hirdey (heart)	Shiva (Gabriel)	Air	Bluish-white (smoky)	Disintegration, decay and death of species	The past, present and future reveal all their secrets
5	Kanth (throat)	Shakti (the Great Mother of the Universe)	Ether (all-pervading)	White (spotless)	The all-controlling power through the three Regents mentioned above with their specific functions	Enables one to become a yogishwar and knower of the Vedas, and to live a life of a thousand years
6	Aggya or Ajna (located behind and between the eyebrows with Antahkaran or the mind)	Atman — the disembodied spirit freed from all raiments	The active life principle; the very soul of Creation	Radiance and Luminosity in full splendor, ineffable	All in all, immanent in everything, the Alpha and Omega of all that is, visible and invisible	Confers the highest gift possible, with all powers, both natural and supernatural

(b) *Svadhishtana* (Hypogastric Plexus) with a six-petaled lotus, extending on four sides plus one below and the other above.

(c) *Manipuraka* (Solar Plexus) with an eight-petaled lotus, having four additional sides in between the original four sides.

(d) *Anahata* (Cardiac Plexus) with a twelve-petaled lotus. It is a lotus of the unstruck sound as the name denotes.

(e) *Vishuddha* (Pharyngeal Plexus) with a sixteen-petaled lotus, being an all-pervasive ethereal lotus. It is a center of great purity as the name indicates.

(f) *Aggya* (Cavernous Plexus) with a two-petaled lotus, also called *Ajna Chakra,* meaning the center of command.

Besides the above plexuses, there is the *Antahkaran* (consisting of *chit, manas, budhi* and *ahankar*), with a lotus of four petals, thus making in all fifty-two petals, corresponding to the fifty-two letters of the alphabet in Sanskrit, the mother of all languages. We have, however, to rise above all *Akshras* to a state beyond called *Neh-akhshra para,* which is eternal and ever-abiding and of which Kabir says:

> *The three lokas and the fifty-two letters*
> *are one and all subject to decay,*
> *But the eternal and the everlasting*
> *holy Word is quite distinct from them.*
>
> KABIR

Each of the two plexuses (see chart on page 65) together make a *granthi* or a tie and these are: *Brahma Granthi, Vishnu Granthi* and *Shiva Granthi.*

The path of the yogins as described above is concerned with meditation at these six centers, beginning from the lowest and gradually rising from one to the next higher by means of pratyahara and dharna as already explained. In this process, one also calls to his aid the *kundalini shakti,* or the great serpentine power lying dormant in three and a half folds in the vagus nerve, in a coiled state like a serpent. This latent energy or power is awakened with the help of pranayam. A yogin tries to collect together all the vital airs in the body at the center of the navel plexus and in this process awakens the latent power as well. From the *Ajna Chakra* he takes hold of the *anahat* sound and reaches *Sahasrar,* the highest heaven of the yogins. It is quite a long, tedious, and difficult path. At each of the centers, one has to work hard for years before one can successfully subdue and pierce through it and ascend to the next higher center. One cannot take to this arduous discipline without a strong and robust physique, capable of withstanding a sustained and strenuous effort for a long time.

As a preliminary step, a yogin has to cleanse the Augean stables with herculean strength and for this, recourse is to be had to *hatha-yoga-kriyas,* or exercises like *dhoti, basti, neoli, gaj karam* and *vajroli,* etc., with a strict diet control. Again, for the control of the mind, he has to take to pranayam or well-regulated breathing exercises such as *puraka, kumbhaka, rechaka* and *sunyaka,* all of which require great care, attention and skill, under the guidance of an adept.

The yoga process, as described above, is fraught with in-numerable difficulties. It is a process akin to that of controlled death, a forcible extraction not only of the spirit current from one center to the other, but of the pranas as well, which makes it all the more difficult. It actually follows the process of dying, being the reversal of the life current as it descends from center to center, in the process of creation. In the death process, the earth element rises up from guda chakra to the indri chakra and gets dissolved in the water there, thus rendering hands and feet lifeless. When the water element rises up to the nabhi chakra, it is transformed into a vaporous state by the fire at the navel region and the generative organ gets paralyzed; next, the fire element itself gets extinguished in the air element at the heart plexus, rendering the region below the heart stark cold. When the air element gets etherealized at the kanth, the seat of the ether, it renders the heart and the pulse motionless. (It may be pointed out that under this system, heart failure does not mark the end of life but only precedes it.) Even in the practice of the Sehaj yogic system, one has to traverse and to follow through exactly the same process, except that the second method is natural, while the first method is deliberate and controlled and therefore extremely difficult to perform. Each of the *tatvas* in turn gets merged in its source; the anna in the pranas, the pranas in the manas, the manas in the vigyan and the vigyan in the kanth plexus. (It may be mentioned that the Vaishnavites and Kabir Panthies wear tulsi leaves and the Shaivites wear shiv-ling around the neck, to remind themselves of the kantha chakra which they set up as their goal.) Instead of this difficult reverse process of yoga from the basic plexus backward and upward to Sahasrar, the region of the thousand-petaled lights, how much easier it would be to ignore the pranas (as we do in our everyday life), collect the sensory current at the seat of the soul at the ajna chakra, where we always are in our awakened state, and move upward straightaway with the help of the Sound Current (to which the yogins gain access after a hard-won battle over the six ganglionic centers in the *pind* or body) to reach Sahasrar. The Sound Current has a magnetic pull, too difficult to resist, when the soul rises above body-consciousness under the guidance of some able and fully competent living Master, capable of awakening the life-impulse within us.

VII. DHYAN (CONTEMPLATION OR MEDITATION)

From continued concentration, as envisaged by dharna, there grows a continuous flow of perception, which is called *dhyan* or contemplation (meditation). Dhyan or meditation is of two kinds: gross and subtle. It is well-nigh impossible to take to subtle meditation all at once. One has therefore to start with gross meditation in the first instance, before taking to the practice of subtle meditation. The gross or objective meditation consists in meditating on the personal aspect of God, *Isht,* a Godman or a Guru (the living Master-saint).

In the subtle meditation, the attention is fixed on the *bindu* or the single eye, the still point in the body behind and between the two eyebrows. It is the intersection of time and the timeless where the Unmanifest becomes manifest. Its reflex is in the *pind* or the lower region of the body, i.e., the *guda chakra,* where lies the coiled energy in a locked up condition. After some practice at the bindu, the dark spot becomes illuminated and gradually the inner light assumes the Radiant Form of the Master. From here begins what is termed the luminous contemplation.

When in meditation, the Godman appears within,
one sees the secrets of Eternity like an open book.

RUMI

While in gross contemplation one meditates on the perceptible form (*swarup*) of the *Isht-deva* or of the Guru, in subtle contemplation one meditates on the *arup* (formless), or the dark point of concentration between the eyebrows, which gradually flowers into radiance.

Here we may sound a note of warning to the seekers after Truth. We cannot have any appreciable results by meditation on the forms of the past Masters who, having discharged their divine mission on earth of contacting *jivas* or souls in their own time, are no longer in touch with the physical world. Again, we have to be on our guard in our search for a perfect Master, for any meditation on the form of an imperfect master will not bear fruit. To avoid all pitfalls, it is much safer to put aside meditation on any form whatsoever, whether of a past or a living Master. It is better that one should carry on the sadhna according to the instructions given, and if the Master is a perfect one, his Radiant Form will of itself appear within and take charge of the individual soul as soon as it rises above body-consciousness. God Himself manifests within in the form of a *Gurudeva* provided of course that the Guru is really embedded in God-power. These remarks apply mutatis mutandis to meditation on *Isht-devas* as is generally done. To meditate on the Formless is beyond human conception, inasmuch as one cannot conceive of the Reality beyond all comprehension. One may in such a case get glimpses of subtle elements, which by themselves cannot lead us anywhere.

The reading of scriptures and other sacred books is not of much avail on this Path except in arousing one's interest. The greatest teacher of mankind is man. It is enough if one knows how to open the pages of the great living book of the human heart ("heart" here signifies the seat of the soul, i.e., *aggya* or *ajna chakra*), which is the only inexhaustible treasure-house of all knowledge and all wisdom. One has simply to close his eyes, withdraw the senses, enter into the sanctuary of his heart and merge his very being into the Supreme Soul in the innermost depths within. He, the Ever-Existent, the Self-Luminous Light, complete in Himself, and eternally the same, dwells in the temple of the human body, and he who wishes to know Him and to reach Him shall have to delve deep within himself, and everything will undoubtedly be revealed to him. "Knock and it shall be opened," is the saying of sages and seers in all times and in all climes. This dip within gives the soul an integral experience of all that exists, whether visible or invisible, a direct intuitive knowledge and divine wisdom, all of which are the gifts that come of themselves, freely and in abundance, if one forgets the world, forgets his friends and relations, forgets his surroundings, nay forgets his very bodily being. Voluntary forgetfulness is the greatest spiritual sadhna. Forgetting all else one must rise above body-consciousness, for this is the primary condition of right meditation.

> Love the Lord thy God with all thy heart, and with all thy soul, and with all thy mind, and with all thy strength.
>
> CHRIST

By deep and silent meditation, one must merge his very being in the sweet contemplation of the Beloved within and lose himself in the Great Soul of the Universe. This is the highest contemplation, and it leads to the most coveted goal of samadhi.

Dhyan as a system of yoga
(the Yoga of Contemplation)

Having considered the essentials of dhyan, we are now in a position to study dhyan as a form of yoga in itself. The mind is all-pervading. Kabir says that manas has its seat in every heart and hence occupies just a middle position in the human system. The mental current is always building its own spheres, and it does so particularly as it descends below. This central position of the mano-mai covering gives it a peculiar importance. It has two sheaths above it, the Vigyan-mai and Anandmai, and two below it, the Pran-mai and Anna-mai. If it turns upward, it gets cognition of wisdom (enlightenment) and bliss. If it turns downward, cognition of the pranic and the physical world.

(i) *Ajna Chakra,* the region of the third eye, behind the two eyebrows, is associated with the anand-mai kosh.

(ii) *Kantha Chakra,* the region between the third eye and the hirdey, is the center of the vigyan-mai kosh.

(iii) *Hirdey Chakra* is the region of the hirdey (heart), where the pranas or the vital airs reign supreme. It is the center of the mano-mai kosh.

(iv) *Nabhi Chakra,* that part of the hirdey region which extends down to the navel, is the center of the pran-mai kosh.

(v) *Indri Chakra,* the region of the navel extending down to guda, is the center of the anna-mai kosh.

(vi) *Guda Chakra* is the basal plexus or the root wherein are rooted all the subtle tubes or nadis.

All the five sheaths (koshas) are the different seats from where one can operate at different levels; the upper two being spiritual, and the lower two being sensory planes.

Anand-mai sheath is the *karan* or the causal body (the seed body) from which everything else below springs, viz., the subtle and the physical planes below. Vigyan-mai is closely associated with and is the nearest to it.

The three sheaths, vigyan-mai, mano-mai and pran-mai, together constitute the *suksham* or the subtle body in man, which is the connecting link between the other two, the anand-mai above, and the anna-mai below, or the causal and the physical, respectively.

The anna-mai kosh is the inner lining, so to say, of the physical body and is closely related to the pran-mai kosh.

In all the three bodies, the mind is the active agent, activated as it is by the life-power of the soul, in the life and light of which it works. To all intents and purposes, the mind power alone is seemingly the force that works and keeps all the other four koshas in order. In the physical body, it is the seat from where the five sensory and five motor powers carry on their operations in the physical plane. Similarly, it is from here (i.e., the mind) that the ten subtle (pranic) powers along with the mental powers of the *chit, manas, budhi* and *ahankar,* carry on their work in the subtle plane. Again, it is the mind which when stilled carries with it all the latent and noumenal impressions and reflects the spirit's light and sound. This then is the vast sway of the mind which extends from the physical to the causal planes, and hence it is often called *Triloki Nath* or the Lord of the three worlds. In the causal plane it serves as a silver screen, which takes and reflects the spiritual vibrations both in the form of Light and Sound.

Advantages of Dhyan Yoga

The advantages of the yoga of contemplation or dhyan are innumerable. One engaged in this form of yoga can by mere contemplation have all his desires fulfilled. "As you think, so you become," is a well-known aphorism. By contemplation on the attributes of God one can develop these attributes within one's own self and be a witness and a testifier to Heaven's Light, while his senses acquire transcendental powers. The mind also tastes of the bliss of *vigyan,* when the *chit vritis,* or the mental modulations, are stilled.

This yoga rids one of all sins, and one feels an inner bliss and halcyon calm. All kinds of mental maladies like fear, shame, vacillation and self-assertiveness, disappear gradually and give place to fearlessness, confidence, firmness and happiness, and one acquires an evenness of temper in all the varying conditions of life. He is not obsessed either by attachment or detachment, and like a lotus flower, floats above and over the slime of common existence. With the knowledge of the true values of life, he grows firm in his convictions and is no longer a prey to the groundless fears and chance winds that blow over him. He has no cause for praise or blame and as such, talks little and does much; all of his acts are motivated by kindliness and good will toward all. His words are honey-sweet and authoritative. He is not tormented by pride and prejudice, but leads a life of perfect moderation and justice. He conquers indolence and idleness; eats little and sleeps little and there is hardly any difference in his state of wakefulness and slumber.

He is ever the same throughout, with a radiant and a beaming face that bespeaks his inner glory. Kabir says:

The world is but a fictitious bondage,
and Kabir centered in the Naam is forever free.

VIII. SAMADHI

The term *samadhi* is derived from two Sanskrit roots: *sam* with its English equivalent "syn" means "together with," and *adhi* (the Primal Being) with its Hebrew equivalent of *Adon* or *Adonai* which denotes "Lord," the two together, *sam* plus *adhi*, denoting a state in which the mind is completely absorbed in the Lord or God. It is a state in which all limiting forms drop away and the individual, with his individuality all dissolved, experiences the great truth—*Ayam Athma Brahma* —"I am Thou."

It is the last and culminating stage in the long-drawn-out process of experimental yoga, and may therefore be said to be the efflorescence of the yogic system. The dhyan itself gradually develops into samadhi when the contemplator or the meditator loses all thought of himself, and the mind becomes *dhya-rupa,* the very form of his thought. In this state the aspirant is not conscious of any external object save of Consciousness itself, a state of all Bliss or perfect happiness.

There are two means through which the state of samadhi may be attained. The *Vedehas* (or those who rise above body-consciousness), achieve it by destroying the very nature of the mind-stuff which runs after material objects all the time, by channelizing it to a one-pointed attention inward. The others develop this state by practicing in the first instance discernment and discrimination through faith, energy and memory. There are other variations of samadhi as well.

In dhyan or meditation (one-pointed attention), one retains the distinction between the contemplator and the contemplated, but in samadhi, or identification with the totality, even these disappear, for one's own individuality is, so to say, anni-hilated. It is this absorption into the Infinite that gives libera-tion from all finitizing adjuncts, for then one gets an insight into the very heart of things and has an experience of the subtle (*adhi-devaka*) and the abstract (*adhi-atmic*) aspects of all that exists.

Samadhi, or identification with the Absolute, may be ac-companied with consciousness of one's individuality, in which case it is known as *savikalpa*, or it may not be accompanied with any such consciousness and is then known as *nirvikalpa*. The former was compared by Sri Ramakrishna to a cotton doll which when put in water gets saturated with it, and the latter to a doll of salt which when immersed in water dis-solves and loses itself in it. Of these, nirvikalpa is clearly the higher, for savikalpa, though it greatly widens one's vision, is yet only a preliminary step toward the unconditioned state. Not all yogins can achieve nirvikalpa, and those that do attain it generally do so only once in their life. They thereby finally escape the realm of name and form and become liberated souls. Their unfructified karmas, both past and present (*san-chit* and *kriyaman*) can no longer bind them, but the momen-tum of their present lives (*prarabdha*) must be completed and must be lived to the very end. On returning from nirvi-kalpa, or the unconditioned state, to everyday human con-sciousness, they live and move as other human beings. But while engaged in worldly duties, they are forever centered in the Divine and are never separate from It. This state of normal activity on the plane of the senses but imbued with God-realization, is designated as *Sehaj Samadhi* or the state of Easy Union.

> *Whether sitting, standing or walking about,*
> *They ever remain in a state of eternal equipoise.*
>
> KABIR

We may also mention yet another form of samadhi, called *Bhava Samadhi,* in which the devotee, lost in devotional music and singing, loses all thought of himself and the world around. This form of samadhi is easy to attain for those of an emotional temperament and affords momentary ecstasy and inner mental relief, but it does not give at-one-ment with the Divine or expand one's consciousness. As such, the term *samadhi* is only loosely applied to it, for it displays none of the central attributes of the super-conscious state, nor is it therefore of much help on the inner spiritual journey.

The state of samadhi is not a stone-like, inert state, or a state of withdrawal similar to that of a tortoise withdrawing into its shell. Each one of us is endowed with a rich inner life, full of untold spiritual gems of which ordinarily we are not conscious in the work-a-day present life of the senses that we usually lead. We can turn inward and expand our vision so as to embrace within its fold not only a cosmic life but even a super-cosmic life as well, extending into vistas beyond the human ken. It is a state of being, a direct perception, an integral experience of the soul, an immediate and direct knowledge of spiritual *anubhava* (inner realization), as it is generally called. Professor Bergson, a great philosopher, believed and felt that there was a higher source of knowledge than intellect, which is confined to ratiocination or the reasoning process. He called it intuition, but this state of being goes even beyond intuition to direct and to immediate knowledge, for intuition is only another name for the sum total of one's past experiences. An ordinary man does not have to reason or intuit about the sun in order to believe in its existence. It is there before him, it is *prataksha* and that renders all proof unnecessary. "All true knowledge exists by itself and is quite independent of the senses. It is the action of the soul and is perfect without the senses . . ." says Ben Jonson. "The surest way into Truth," says Henri Bergson, "is by perception, by intuition, by reasoning to a certain point, then by taking a mortal leap." It is *divya drishti* or *jnana chakshu* (i.e., direct experience of the soul, of the Reality Itself). It is through spiritual flashes and glimpses from beyond that one gets some view of Truth in the form of spiritual insight, inspiration and revelation. The spiritual experience, though it stands by itself and is beyond the farthest limits of reason, does not however contradict reason, but makes reason perfect.

Again, samadhi is *chaitanya* or all-consciousness, as distinguished from *jar* samadhi. A Hatha yogin, by the practice of Khechari Mudra, withdraws his pranas into the Sahasrar Chakra, the seat of the jiva-atma or soul, and can sit in a mountain cave or underground cavity in this state of inanity for months and years. This is a kind of *yoga nidra* or yogic sleep, and does not give any super-sensory knowledge or spiritual experience. As opposed to this, one who is in chaitanya samadhi is in a state of perfect awareness and can come out of it at will with a new supra-mental experience and spiritual wisdom. In jar samadhi, one cannot break the samadhi by oneself and others have to do it by a complicated procedure of massages, etc. A Raja yogin, a Bhakta or a Jnana yogin, can be awakened easily by someone merely shaking his body, or by blowing a conch or striking a gong. This chaitanya samadhi is achieved when the gunas, devoid of motion, become dormant and the power of consciousness gets established in its own nature; hence it is often termed as *kaivalya* samadhi or a samadhi of perfect ease and independence.

Samadhi Yoga

Yoga, as said elsewhere, means steadiness of mind, born of chit-vriti-nirodha (nullification of mind or elimination from the mind of all mental vibrations), and the term *samadhi,* comprising the two Sanskrit roots *sam* and *adhi,* denotes acceptance, absorption, steadiness in contemplation, or deep inward concentration.

Each individual comes into the world with a background of his own, which fits him for a particular type of yoga. He should therefore engage in such yogic practices as may be best suited to him. Samadhi Yoga is the highest form of yoga. Some children are naturally prone to it, and some persons can take to it directly without even going through the hard discipline usually enjoined for the general run of people. Its practice can, in such cases, be prescribed without any scruples to those ripe for it through past *samskaras*.

The mind gets *vigyan* or *jnana* in the plexus of the throat (*Kanth Chakra*), which is closely associated with the seat of consciousness in a waking state. The *vigyan* and the *anand* or consciousness of bliss dawns only in *Sahasrar* or *Sahas-dal-Kanwal*, the thousand-petaled lotus behind the two eyebrows, and Samadhi Yoga aims at the realization of this state wherein one may consciously feel the inherent bliss of the soul. Samadhi then is the state of unalloyed bliss, which is the direct source of everything else: *vigyan* (*jnana*), *manas* (the mind-stuff), *pranas* (the vital airs), and *anna* (the physical world of sense objects). *Anand* or bliss is the intrinsic and basic substratum of all that exists, and this is why there is an innate craving in all creatures for satiety, happiness and bliss. Not to speak of man, even the animals, the insects, and in fact all created beings, are ever in search of it in varying degrees and aspects, each according to its own nature. But its full significance or consciousness dawns only on man when in a state of samadhi. It is a gradual process of rising from one plane to another, until *jnana* is united with bliss at the level of samadhi and one consciously and fully realizes the blissful state. This is the sole end and aim of Samadhi Yoga.

The essential quality of bliss is the characteristic of the soul or atman. It is the veil of *vigyan* or *jnana* that covers their blissful condition. The moment this veil is removed and one rises above the higher level of the intellect (self-consciousness), one realizes true happiness and the blissful sea of the atman spreading in and around him to measureless depths and to immeasurable heights. All the intermediary four koshas: *anna, prana, manas,* and *vigyan,* are but wayside halts on the spiritual journey for working out step by step, the yogic sadhna to its full efflorescence or *jnana,* and provide nourishment to consciousness as it descends lower. But when it once becomes steady and contacts the spiritual bliss, it becomes aware of the true and higher values of life, ceases to interest itself in the passing and shadowy pleasures of the world, and seeks absorption in Absolute Bliss. This is the culminating point in the spiritual sadhna or practice and when it is achieved, there remains nothing else to be done. But the trouble with most of us is that we often come to regard *jnana* or *gyan* as the goal of all human endeavors and therefore do not attempt to pierce through its veil and go beyond into the consciousness of the self and taste of the blissful fountainhead of the soul that lies ahead. The result is that without contact with, and a foretaste of, the awareness of bliss, we become *vachak gyanis* or *gyanis* only in name, ever a prey to groundless fears and depressing states of mind, doubts and distress, which may assail us in the work-a-day life in the world. It is therefore rightly said that:

"A real *jnani* is one who communes with the Word."

Vigyan is, after all, a state below that of *anand* or Real Bliss. As worshipers of the physical body remain entangled in the web of *anna-mai kosha,* those of the sensuous pleasures in the network of *pran-mai kosha* and the mind-ridden in the *mano-mai kosha,* so do many so-called *jnanis* or *gyanis* remain caught in the quagmire of *vigyan-mai kosha,* without realizing that there is still a stage beyond and above it, and of far greater importance. The four enshrouding sheaths are thick and heavy, folds within folds, and cover up the crest jewel of perfect bliss (*anand*). The great jeweller, God, has kept *anand* hidden in the innermost and enchanting casket of *vigyan* which, with its colorful witchery, keeps even the so-called *jnani* bound to body-consciousness.

The wrestlers, the body builders and the *charvakas* or epicureans, who regard physical well-being and pleasure as the goal of life, belong to the class of *anna-mai jivas,* who live and die for this cause alone. Next, there are persons who are a little bold, courageous and enterprising. They nourish their ideas, principles and convictions as well as their physical forms and are ever ready to stand by them, even at times at the cost of worldly comforts. Such persons are *pran-mai jivas,* for they are swayed by the pranas, on which all life depends, and they have in them the preponderance of the water element, for prana means life and life is the outcome of water. In the Chhandogya Upanishad it is said that water and not food is the source of life, and it is on water that life depends. Again, persons endowed with strong emotions and feelings remain constantly attached more to manas than to anything else, for in them the element of fire predominates. All poets, writers, inventors, designers and architects come under the category of *mano-mai jivas.* All their energy is channeled in the direction of the mind and they engage in pursuits near to their heart. They are martyrs to the path of the mind. Next, we have a class of persons who, while caring reasonably for their bodily comforts, and for their thoughts and beliefs and mental pursuits, are in the main wedded to intellectual reasoning or ratiocination in finding out the why and wherefore of things. They are classified as *vigyan-mai jivas* and are swayed mostly by the air element in them. The highest in the scale of human creation are the *anand-mai jivas* who give preference to Bliss and true happiness above everything else, are ever engaged in search of it, and do not rest until they

find it out and live by it. They are ethereal beings and live
in the all-pervading ether with no limitations. It is the most
suble of the enveloping sheaths, beyond which lies the state
of *Nirvana* itself, perpetual bliss untrammeled by any *koshas,* ineffably serene, a sublime state of conscious rest in
Omniscience.

3. Ashtang Yoga and Modern Man

This then is the long and the short of the yoga system as
originally propounded by Hiranyagarbha, and expounded to
the world by Gaudapada and Patanjali, the well-known philosophers and thinkers. In these few pages, an attempt has
been made to give a brief account of the yoga philosophy as
it has come down to us from the hoary past, and which is
still considered the keystone of the ancient wisdom of India.

The yoga system is a discipline involving intense and solitary meditation coupled with physical exercises and postures
to discipline and control the mind and the pranas, so as to
make them run in a particular manner that may help in
subduing the senses. As such, it is meant for the purification
of the body and mind, and prepares the way for the beatific
vision. Devotion to God or *Ishwara* also plays an important
part in the yogic realization. The personal God of the yoga
philosophy stands apart in the yoga system because the final
goal for some of the yogins is the separation of atman from
the mind and not union with God. This system, therefore,
always works in the domain of dualism. Its principal aim is
the separation of the layered *jiva* from the embodied state so
as to become *atman,* freed from the conditioned state of
mind and matter. Both the understanding will and the oscil-
lating mind then stop their individual working and become
stilled, thus liberating the soul to shine in its own true and
native light.

The yogic exercises generally yield health, strength and longevity, and help to a certain extent in defying disease, decay and early death. One may also acquire psychic and supernatural powers by controlling Nature and Nature's laws. By the heightened power of the senses, the yogins can hear from and see at long distances, penetrate into the past and the present and even into the future, transmit thoughts and perform miracles.

Many modern scholars, more so those with Western modes of thought, have, when first confronted by yoga, tended to dismiss it as no more than an elaborate means of self-hypnotism. Such an attitude is quite unscientific even though it often parades under the garb of science. It is generally the result of prejudice born of ignorance or a superficial knowledge of the subject. It is natural for us to attempt to relegate to the realm of superstition, phenomena with which we are unfamiliar and which defy our habitual ways of thought about life, for to study them, to understand them, to test and accept them, would require effort and perseverance of which most of us are incapable. It is not unlikely that some so-called yogins may justify the label of "self-hypnotists." But those few who genuinely merit the name of yogins are too humble to court publicity and have nothing about them to suggest the neurotic escapist. They invariably display a re-markably sensitive awareness to life in all its complexity and variety, and this awareness coupled with their humility makes all talk of self-delusion quite inapt, irrelevant and even ridic-ulous. For, to seek the Unchanging behind the changing, the Real behind the phenomenal, is certainly not to "hyp-notize" oneself. If anything, it displays a spirit of enquiry that is exceptional in its honesty and integrity, that is content with nothing less than the absolute truth, and the kind of renunciation it demands is most difficult to practice. Hence it is, that as time passes, as knowledge is gradually undermining ignorance, the former philistinism is steadily wearing away. The new developments of the physical sciences have had no small share in furthering this process, for by revealing that everything in this physical universe is relative and that matter is not matter per se but ultimately a form of energy, it has confirmed, at the lower level of the yogic concept at least, the conception of the world inherent in the yogic sys-tem, giving it a scientific validity which was earlier doubted.

Nevertheless, even if one accepts the basis of Ashtang Yoga as it has come down to us from Patanjali, one must confess that it is far from easy to practice. Even Gaudapada admitted that to pursue it was like attempting to empty the sea drop by drop with the aid of a blade of grass. Hence it was that even when it was first developed it demanded a highly rigorous discipline of life, and the ideal of the four *ashramas* was the inevitable consequence. If one was to achieve any-thing substantial, one had to begin from infancy itself. The first twenty-five years of *brahmcharya* were to be utilized in the proper development of one's body and mind, in building up physical and spiritual health capable of withstanding life's rigors. The next twenty-five years, *grehastya,* were to be lived as a householder, as the head of a family, a prop to the old, a supporter to the wife, and a sound teacher to the children. Obligations to society performed, death drawing nearer, and life tasted to the full, one was free to seek its inner meaning and ripe for its understanding. And so, the succeeding twenty-five years were to be spent in *vanprasth,* in the solitude of mountain and forest, until through various sadhnas and strenuous meditation one had gained enlighten-ment. Now at last one was fit to be called a *sanyasin* and able to devote the last quarter of the century-span as envisaged in the perfect life, to the task of assisting one's fellow men in their search for spiritual freedom.

Even in olden days, the ideal of the four *ashramas* was

not an easy one. Little wonder then that yoga was restricted to the chosen few and was not propagated as a course to be followed by the common people, continuing only as a mystery school whose torch was passed on from *guru* to *chela* (*sadhak*) in a restricted line. If anything, modern conditions have rendered its pursuit in this form even more difficult and well-nigh impossible. As life has become more complex and the various professions more specialized, men no longer find it possible to devote the first twenty-five years of their life solely to the cultivation of body and mind in preparation for the final quest. They must spend them in schools, colleges and institutes, which employ most of their resources in training them for a career. Nor, with the ever-growing population, is it feasible to expect one-fourth of the members of society—*grehastis*—to provide the means of physical sustenance for the remaining three-quarters, as was once perhaps possible.

As if this were not enough, the integrated eightfold yoga of Patanjali seems to have grown more specialized and complicated with the passage of time. Each of its branches has developed to a point where it almost seems a complete subject in itself. Little wonder then that man, practicing in their various details the various yamas and niyamas, or mastering the different asanas or learning to control the pranic or mansic (mental) energies, begins to imagine that his particular field of specialization is not, as Patanjali envisaged, just a rung in the ladder of the integrated yoga, but yoga itself. No doubt, he derives some benefit or other from whatever he practices, often acquiring uncanny psychic or physical powers; but these very gifts, by distracting his attention from the ultimate goal, become a positive hindrance to real progress instead of being aids to it. Only a very few men of exceptional physical endurance, long life and an extradordinary capacity for not forgetting the distant goal, can, in our time, pursue Patanjali's Ashtang Yoga to its logical conclusion, its highest purpose: at-one-ment with Brahman. For the rest, it must remain either too difficult to practice, or a process that, by encouraging them to mistake the intermediate for the final, the means for the end, defeats its own purpose.

If spirituality must entail a slow ascension through all the rungs of this intricate and involved ladder of yoga, then it cannot choose but remain a closed secret to mankind at large. If, however, it is to become a free gift of Nature like the sun, the air and the water, then it must make itself accessible through a technique which places it within the reach of all, the child no less than the adult, the weak no less than the strong, the householder no less than the *sanyasin*. It is of such a technique that Kabir and Nanak gave us hope and will be dealt with later.

CHAPTER THREE

The Forms of Yoga

H AVING discussed the yoga system in general as expounded by Patanjali, we will now proceed to study the various forms of yoga that arose subsequently. Beginning with the traditional, we are told of four distinct types: (1) Mantra Yoga, (2) Hatha Yoga, (3) Laya Yoga and (4) Raja Yoga. Most of these draw heavily on Patanjali and present reformulaations of his basic teachings, each specializing in one or another of its aspects. As such, some degree of repetition is unavoidable; yet we must risk it, if only to have a clearer view of the vast subject of yoga.

I. Mantra Yoga or the Yoga of Utterance

They even forget, that all deities reside in the human breast.

WILLIAM BLAKE

Mantra Yoga is concerned, in the main, with the acquisition of one or the other material or mental power or powers through the constant repetition of a particular *mantra* or oral formula in order to attract the presiding power or deity to which the mantra relates, and then to press that power into service, good or bad, according to the will and pleasure of the practitioner. One who uses these powers for effecting evil and doing harm to others often runs the risk of self-immolation and usually falls a prey to the wrath of the deity concerned. Those who employ such powers for selfish motives with the object of material gains to themselves at the cost of

86

THE FORMS OF YOGA

others, very soon lose their power, and in the end ruin them-selves. These powers may, however, be profitably used for the good of others and there is not much harm in that, though it may mean loss of some vital energy after each such act. All types of miracles of the lowest order, like thought-reading, thought-transference, faith-healing, particularly in cases of nervous and mental diseases, fall under this category. It is therefore much better to avoid such things and to conserve whatsoever psychic powers one may acquire, and use them for gaining at least the lower spiritual planes and regions which form the seat of the deities concerned, in a spirit of selfless devotion. Then all the psychic powers will of themselves function without incurring any loss by one's own acquisition of them. It should however be borne in mind that repetition of the mantras per se does not bear any fruit unless it is done with full attention fixed on the specific mantras, and with intense devotion such as may set up par-ticular vibrations connected therewith. But Mantra Yoga by itself is not of any value in self-realization, and more often than not those who practice this form of yoga remain ever entangled in useless pursuits of one kind or another as de-scribed above, with no great benefit to themselves in the upliftment of the self or soul.

As regards the exercise of *mantra siddhis* or supernatural powers acquired through the efficacy of meditation on man-tras, Patanjali, in his *Yog Sutras,* sounds a definite note of warning:

> *They are obstacles to samadhi, powers but in worldly state.*

Technique in Mantra Yoga

Mantra Yoga is the yoga of rhythmic repetition of her-metically sealed formulas—sacred and secret—prepared by the ancient *mantrakaras* (adepts in phonetics and in the power of sounds, including supersonics or sounds beyond the human ken), each designed separately for winning over the particular god or goddess representing one or the other powers of Nature. It may be practised with or without the aid of a rosary of *Rudrakhsha,* as the Shaivites do, or of Tulsi beads, as used by the Vaishnavites.

The mantras represent vibrations. The most sacred of the Vedic mantras is that of the *Gayatri.* It is the *mool mantra* of the Vedas and hence is considered to be of the first importance. Its virtue is said to be great and its japa or repetition has been enjoined on all Hindus from a very early age. The easiest and the most efficacious is the sacred syllable AUM, symbolizing the creative life-principle itself, and hence most of the mantras themselves begin with this sacred syllable. The Advaitists, who see the power of God immanent in all forms and as all-pervading, believe in the mantra of identification of atman with Parmatman: *Aham Braham Asmi* (I am Brahman), and *Ayam Athma Brahman* (I am Thou); and these are often shortened into *Soham* or *Sohang* and *Hansa* or *Aham-sah,* meaning respectively "I am He" and "He is I." The Vedantists repeat *Om Tat Sat* (Aum is the Truth and the Reality) and the Buddhists *Om Mani Padme Hum.* Next in the scale are mantras dedicated or addressed to this or that deity in adoration, praise, propitiation or entreaty for boons.

The efficacy of a mantra depends on its right pronunciation, right appreciation of its significance, which is often very profound, the right attitude of the person engaged in Mantra Yoga, and on the competence of the preceptor or Guru, who has mastered not only the technique but has successfully manifested for himself the seed-power lying hidden in the core of the mantra, and can offer it as a *prasad* or a gift of grace to his disciple.

Some of the mantras bring forth quick results, some fructify in their own good time and some bear fruit according to the merit of the individual concerned. Some are, however, of a forbidden type and hence inimical in nature, and more often than not they prove harmful.

Again, the effect of a mantra also depends on how the japa is performed. The japa done in whispers is considered as more meritorious than the one uttered loudly, and japa done in low murmurs is still better, while *mansic japa* done with the tongue of thought is the most meritorious.

The japas too are of different kinds according to the occasion, the season and intention of the doer. The *nitya japas* are, for example, to be performed every day as a matter of routine. The *namittika* are for certain ceremonial occasions. The *prayashchitta* are those done as a penance, atoning for lapses from the path of rectitude. Then there are *chala* and *achala* japas, that can be performed at any time, at any place, and under any circumstances, in any state or position. The others require a specific asana, place, time and direction, etc., coupled with a regular and elaborate ritual, e.g., offerings of flowers, scent, incense, light-waving and bell-tinkling, *havan* and *tarpan* (rituals of fire and water), with various purificatory acts.

For success in Mantra Yoga it is necessary that the sadhak should observe purity within and without, having a full-hearted devotion, exemplary character and conduct, before he can have any degree of concentration and contemplation.

We observe similar practices among the Muslim faqirs, who practice *vird* or repetition of sacred words like *Hu, Haq, Analhaq,* and use a *tasbih* (rosary) for the purpose. The Christian monks also tell their beads and chant hymns and psalms.

II. HATHA YOGA

This form of yoga deals with the control of the body and the bodily activities as the means of stilling the mind. Its aim

is to make the human body strong and capable enough to
stand and endure the hardest and the toughest conditions, and
to make it immune, as far as possible, from physical diseases
and ailments. But beyond a robust physique and possible longevity through the practice of pranayam or *habs-i-dam,* as it
is called by the Muslims (control and regulation of breath),
it is not of much help in self-realization by itself, though it
may to a certain extent prepare the ground for a higher type
of spiritual discipline leading thereto. It is in a sense a "ladder
to Raja Yoga." It cannot even give the mind any great degree
of control, as it is commonly supposed to do. By practicing
Hatha Yoga, one may come to gain some siddhis or psychic
powers through the exercise of certain asanas, mudras and
bandhas, or physical positions and postures, and the practice
of pranayam. The system includes observance of a number of
penances and ascetic austerities like fasts and vigils, *maun* or
a vow of silence for months and years, *panch agni tapas*
(sitting with lighted fires on four sides and the burning sun
overhead), standing on one leg, suspending oneself with head
downward, etc. Some of the Christian saints went to great
extremes like the wearing of nail-studded tunics, horsehair
shirts, scourging of the body, self-flogging, all in imitation of
the sufferings of Christ. Even among the Muslim *shias,* we see
the traces of self-torture, when during the *Muharram* days,
they beat their breasts and backs with knives fastened to iron
chains in commemoration of the terrible sufferings that Hassan
and Hussain, the grandsons of the Prophet, had to undergo
along with a handful of their faithful followers, at the hands
of their co-religionists under Yazid, on the burning plains of
Karbla in defense of their faith. But all these terrible self-
chastisements, however heroic in themselves, hardly grant any
spiritual benefit. Of what good is it to torture and torment
the body, when the serpent of the mind lies safely hid far
beneath the surface and continues to thrive unscathed?

Leaving aside such forms of self-torture, the Hatha Yoga proper aims at perfecting the body as an instrument for higher types of yogas, and as such may have some value, to enable the body to stand the stress and strain involved in them. But even the routine of *Hatha Yoga Kriyas* is too difficult to perform, and often leads to inner complications which at times prove serious and incurable and endanger life.

These kriyas are meant for purification of the arteries and other channels in the body of all kinds of accumulated mineral deposits like chalk, lime and salt, etc., which clog the system and are the root-cause of decay and disease. This process of deintoxication and rejuvenation is done by means of purificatory acts called *Shat Karma* (meaning six acts), which are:

(i) *Neti Karma* (cleaning of the nose): A piece of thin muslin about three-fourths yard long is twisted into a string-like form and covered with a coating of wax. It is passed through each of the nostrils in turn and taken out of the mouth after a little rubbing so as to clean them of phlegm, etc. It is helpful in curing diseases of the nose and throat. It keeps the head cool, and improves the sight. Those suffering from nose and eye disorders or acidity may substitute for it *jala neti,* or douching the nasal channels with pure water.

(ii) *Dhoti Karma* (washing the stomach): A long piece of cloth three inches in width and measuring about seven yards in length is soaked in tepid water and then slightly wrenched. It is gradually swallowed down the throat into the stomach with the help of warm water, keeping about two feet of the other end in hand. After retaining it for a few minutes and shaking the abdomen, it is taken out very, very slowly. It cleanses the alimentary canal of impurities like mucus, bile and phlegm and cures an enlarged spleen and a cough, etc. This practice requires extreme care and attention so that the cloth may not get entangled in the intestines and result in serious complications, which might even prove fatal. It should not be practiced when suffering from inflammation of the throat and bronchial disorders, irritation of the stomach or during coughing, etc.

(iii) *Basti Karma* (washing the bowels): It is a kind of enema whereby water is drawn in through the rectum into the lower intestines. After retaining it for some time, it is churned sideways and thrown out. It removes constipation and ejects inner, hardened refuse matter, which generally keeps sticking to the inside. An addition of a little glycerine to the tepid water makes it more beneficial. It is used for ailments connected with the male organ and the anus and it cures gaseous disorders of bile or lymph, and diseases of the spleen and liver. A daily resort to Basti weakens the tender intestines and may inflame the inner surface, and hence the need for careful guidance in such matters. It may be substituted by air cleansing if necessary, by drawing in and letting out air instead of water.

(iv) *Gaja Karni* or *Kunj Karma*: It is also known as *Shankha Pashala*. The practice consists in taking a bellyful of water and then swilling it within by muscular activity and throwing it out from the mouth as a gaja or elephant does with his trunk. In this way two or three quarts of warm water are taken and vomited out after washing the inner system by a circulatory motion of the muscles within. It is particularly useful for those who suffer from biliousness or acidity.

(v) *Niyoli Karma* (shaking the belly): It is done by sitting erect in Siddha or Padma Asana with hands settled on the knees. The upper part of the body along with the intestines is then to be churned or shaken rapidly from right to left so as to remove all inner impurities adhering to the inner walls. This practice is useful in ridding one of abdominal ailments of gastric and gaseous nature by releasing the digestive secretions. It helps in muscular contractions which in turn aid yogic breathing or pranayam.

(vi) *Tratak Karma* (gaze fixing) : It is a *dristi sadhna* and consists in fixing the gaze, first on external centers, and then gradually on inner centers as explained at some length in the foregoing pages dealing with Yog Vidya and Yog Sadhna, in the section on "pranayam." By it, the gazing faculty becomes steady and when turned inward, one begins to see the wonders of the inner world of Trikuti, the highest heaven of such yogins.*

Besides the above, there are two other practices:

(i) *Kalpal Dhoti* (rapid breathing in and out) for purification of the lungs. It can conveniently take the place of Neti, but should be avoided in the rainy season and in ill-health. The breathing should be quick but not too fast, so that it may not affect the lungs and the respiratory system.

(ii) *Shankh Pashali* : It consists in taking water by mouth and immediately evacuating it through the rectum after a little shaking of the abdomen. It cleanses the entire digestive system by washing it clean of all impurities.

---

* Baba Garib Das tells us that the yogins regard Til as *Kshar*, Sahansdal Kamal or Sahasrar as *Akshar* and Trikuti as *Neh-Akshar*. The yogishwars go a step further and starting from Sahasrar, they go into Daswan Duar while the saints' nomenclature in this respect is Trikuti for Kshar, Daswan Duar for Akshar and Bhanwar Gupha for Neh-Akshar, and then the beyond, i.e., Sat Lok.

In the scriptures, Akshar stands for the creative life-principle and it is said that one who knows and realizes its essence qualifies for the path Godward. The *Akshar Purush* with the help of *Anhad* or unending Sound Principle is responsible for the creation of the astral and physical planes below Trikuti. These are subject to dissolution, and are known as Kshar as opposed to Akshar, the indestructible *Kutastha* and *Avyakt* (above decay and dissolution). Beyond Kshar and Akshar is the *Purshottam* or *Paramatma* (the Oversoul God). Cf. Bhagavad Gita 12:3-4 and 15:16-17.

The spiritual regions beyond Trikuti are upheld by *Sat-Shabda* (*Sphota* or the Word-essence) and the lord of these divisions is Neh Akshar but he too cannot outlive the grand dissolution. The Sat Lok or Muqam-i-Haq is the first Grand Division that lies beyond the border line of the dissolution and it is eternally the same (*Neh-Akshar-Para*) and this in fact is the abode of the saints, it being their native homeland.

All these processes, if not done under the direction, guidance and control of an adept in the yogic sadhnas, more often than not do more harm than good. It must be admitted that there is something artificial and unnatural about them, and cases have been reported wherein even adepts have suffered from their performance. It is therefore better to take recourse to natural ways of simple, wholesome and fresh vegetarian diet in its natural state, some cow's milk and ghee, fresh water, regular but untiring exercises, deep breathing, etc., all of which are free from any of the dangers attending the Hatha Yoga practices.

Thus we see that in Hatha Yoga one has, in the first instance, to set the physical house in order, and that this is done by the practice of Shat Karmas, or the six preliminary practices as described above. After this, for successfully working out this type of yoga and acquiring proficiency therein, recourse is to be had to the following disciplines:

(a) Scrupulous cultivation of yamas and niyamas.

(b) Observance of *sanjam,* or moderation and discipline, in all phases of life, and particularly in thoughts, words and deeds.

(c) Physical postures of asanas, mudras and bandhas.

(d) Pranayam or the control and regulation of the respiratory system, all of which have been explained elsewhere in Ashtang Yoga.

We may now consider what some writers have said regarding the place of Hatha Yoga in the spiritual path. Shri Yogindra, in his Introduction to his *Hatha Yoga (Simplified),* speaks of Hatha Yoga as follows:

The necessity of this system of yoga must have been felt in the ancient past when the discipline and education of the physical became an essential form of discipline and control of the mental, the moral and the psychic. In this context, Hatha Yoga should be, and is, regarded as the methodical approach to the attainment of the highest in yoga. Because it deals primarily with the physical, the human body, in relation to the mental, it has been appropriately identified as the physiological yoga or *Ghatasya Yoga.*

The author Alain Danielou in his book, *Yoga: The Method of Reintegration,* describes the method of Hatha Yoga as reintegration through strength, because "self is not within the reach of the weak," and dealing with its object and method, says:

Hatha Yoga is the name given to the technical practices and disciplines by which the body and the vital energies can be brought under control. Although one of the means of yoga, it is the first preparation toward the way of reintegration, essential for further realization.

All treatises on yoga insist that the sole purpose of the physical practices of Hatha Yoga is to surmount physical obstacles on the spiritual or royal path of reintegration—Raja Yoga.

"Hatha" literally means "will-power," or indomitable will to do a thing or to achieve an object howsoever out of the common run it may appear to be. The meaning of the word "Hatha" Danielou goes on to explain from the *Goraksha Samhita,* as:

The syllable "Ha" represents the sun, and the syllable "tha" represents the moon and the conjunction (yoga) of the sun and moon is therefore Hatha Yoga.

The cosmic principles which manifest themselves in the planetary world as the sun and the moon, are found in every aspect of existence. In man, they appear mainly under two forms, one in the subtle body, the other in the gross body. In the subtle body they appear as two channels along which our perceptions travel between the subtle center at the base of the spinal chord and the center at the summit of the head. These two are called ida and pingala; one corresponding to the cold aspect of the moon and the other to the warm aspect of the sun.

In the gross body, the lunar and solar principles correspond to the respiratory, cool, and the digestive, warm, vital energies, and are called prana and apana. It is by coordinating these two most powerful vital impulses that the yogin achieves his aim. In relation to breath, the cold air breathed in is spoken of as prana vayu and the warm air breathed out as apana vayu.

Hatha Yoga has certain undeniable advantages, many of which have already been described in the previous chapter when discussing asanas, pranayam or pratyahara. It lays the foundation of a healthy life capable of withstanding many physical strains through the elimination of toxic and impure matter within the bodily system. To a yogin, death comes not as the tortured end of a long process of decay, but like the autumn leaf or the ripe fruit, it is the severance that is naturally wrought by inner maturity. Gain of control over various physical functions naturally brings with it some degree of mental control as well, for any rigorous discipline of the body is impossible without a discipline of the will, and the development of the one stimulates the other.

Nevertheless, the physical and psychic powers that Hatha Yoga ensures to the successful sadhak are not without their snares and dangers. Instead of being kept strictly private for further spiritual progress or used only for the most humanitarian purposes, they are often employed for winning public applause and wealth. It is not for nothing that the common man associates this yoga with men who walk on burning charcoals, swallow glass-pieces or metal blades, eat snakeheads and rodents, hold back running cars, or allow themselves to be run over by trucks or elephants. The serious-minded student of yoga, observing this abuse, must use these practices strictly as stepping-stones to Raja Yoga or else discard them altogether as yet another distraction from the goal, another means for pampering the ego which they set out to master. Huston Smith, in *The Religions of Man,* has put the matter roundly:

> Some persons are chiefly interested in coordinating their bodies. Needless to say, they have their Indian counterparts — men who take mastery of the body as their basic interest. . . . Whereas the West has sought strength and beauty, India has been interested in precision and control, ideally complete control over the body's every function . . . Julian Huxley has ventured cautiously that India appears to have discovered some things about what the body can be brought to do of which the West has no inkling. This extensive body of instruction comprises an authentic yoga, Hatha Yoga. Originally it was practiced as a preliminary to spiritual yoga, but as it has largely lost this connection, it need not concern us here. A judgement of the Hindu sages on this matter can be ours as well: incredible things can be done with the body if this is what interests you and you are willing to give your life to it. But these things have little to do with enlightenment. In fact, they grow out of a desire to show off, their mastery makes for pride and so is inimical to spiritual progress.

III. Laya Yoga

This is the yoga of absorption or mergence. *Laya* literally means to lose oneself in some overpowering idea or a ruling passion. By a deep and continued absorption through concentration, one is gradually led to a state of forgetfulness of everything else, including the bodily self, and to having only one thought uppermost in one's mind, which is the objective before him for realization. This obsession may be for anything,

worldly gain, power and pelf, name and fame; even for
acquiring riddhis and siddhis or supernatural powers or, above
all, for attaining the Ultimate Reality we call God. Thus there
are various forms and stages of Laya Yoga, the highest of
course being absorption in the contemplation of God—the
conception of the yogins in this behalf being the astral light
and the means thereto lying through the practice of mudras
or locked postures, many of which have already been described
in the foregoing chapter; for Laya Yoga corresponds closely
to Patanjali's views on dhyan. The highest type of contemplation in Laya Yoga takes one above body-consciousness, leading
to the Divine Ground of the human soul—Sahasrar or the
headquarters of the subtle regions, with a thousand-petaled
lotus full of lights in a pyramidical formation. Forgetfulness of
everything but the subject of continued meditation is the key
to success in this form of yoga. It is the natural result of pratyahara and dharna leading to dhyan, which combined together constitute the foundation of Laya Yoga.

The yogins believe in the twin principles of Purush and
Prakriti, the positive male and the negative female principles,
both in Man and in Nature. In Man this Nature-energy lies
coiled up at the basal root-center in the body, and the process
consists in awakening it into activity by the performance of
asanas and the practice of yogic breathing, and in carrying it
up through the central nadi—sukhman—until it reaches
and merges in the highest center—the Purush in Sahasrar—
and hence the term yoga of mergence. For success in Laya
Yoga, one has to rely on the lights of the various elements that
predominate at the chakras, or centers, in the pind or physical
body. As this journey of mergence of the mind into chid-akash
is not free from risks, it is necessary to work it out under the
strict guidance of an adept in the line.

Laya Yoga differs vitally from other forms of yoga, which
in the main have a positive approach by concentration or con-

templation on some fixed object. In Laya Yoga, the approach
is of a negative type. Instead of controlling the mind as yoga
systems generally do, it concentrates on controlling the Kundalini, the vital energy, which lies hidden and latent, and it is
perhaps because it deals with a latency that it is termed as
Laya Yoga.

IV. RAJA YOGA

As the name indicates and implies, it means "the royal road
to reintegration;" the reintegration of soul which is now in a
state of disintegration, having lost its cohesion through the
diversifying influence of the mind running into so many out-
going channels. This path offers a scientific approach Godward
and is best suited to persons gifted with a scientific mind and
a scientific outlook, both within and without, and given to
experimentation. It is based on the assumption that the true
self in man is quite different from, and more wonderful than,
what it is commonly supposed and appears to be in the work-
a-day life where it is subject to limitations that crowd in and
press upon it from all sides, making it look for all practical
purposes a finite element and not the limitless reality it really
is.

Again, the experiments involved in Raja Yoga are to be
performed on one's own self, unlike those in other sciences, in
which the whole process involved is one of experiment on outside nature. A Raja yogin is not expected to take things for
granted or to blindly accept an authority, scriptural or otherwise. His is essentially a path of self-experiment in the laboratory of the mind, and he proceeds slowly but steadily, step by
step, and never stops until the goal is reached.

Man, according to Raja Yoga, is a "layered entity" and is
clothed in so many folds, one within the other, e.g., body,
bodily habits, mode of life, inherited and acquired, senses and
addictions, vital airs, restless mind with innumerable mental

vibrations, ever-active will and egocentricity, etc., all of which form koshas or veils covering the atman. Within these lies the crest-jewel of Being itself, the ever-abiding Self underneath the phenomenal personality. Thus complete liberation (*mukti*), consists in complete release from the countless finitizing processes enveloping the Infinite Ocean of the Creative Life Principle, so as to· have all power, all life, all wisdom, all joy, all bliss and everything else in its fullness. In other words, it means depersonalization of the soul by literally tearing down the personality or the mask which an actor dons when he comes on to the stage to play his role. The job of a Raja yogin then, is to unmask the reality within him by removing the numberless masks or false identifications, and thereby to separate the great Self from the enshrouding sheaths by which it is encumbered.

Ashtang Yoga or the eightfold path of Patanjali leads to what is commonly known as Raja Yoga. It is the ladder whereby one achieves *Nirbij Samadhi, Unmani, Sehaj-awastha* or the *Turiya pad,* which is the crown of all the yoga systems and the efflorescence of the yogic art. It deals with the training of the mind and its psychic powers to an extent which may lead to Enlightenment, whereby true perception is attained and one gains an equipoise, a state of waking trance. His soul is unshakably fixed inwardly at its center, *sam,* even though he may apparently be engaged in worldly pursuits like the rest of mankind. This state is the pinnacle of all yogic endeavors and practices, and once attained, the yogin, while living in the world, is yet no longer of the world. This is how Raj Rishi Janak and Lord Krishna, the prince of the yogins, lived in the world, ever engaged in worldly pursuits and activities, carrying the wheel of the world in their hands in perpetual motion, yet with a still center fixed in the Divine Plane. All of their actions were characterized by activity in inactivity. Such is the apex in the yoga system, a state in which the senses, the mind and the intellect come to a standstill. In the Katha Upanishad, we have:

> When all the senses are stilled, when the mind is at rest, when the intellect wavers not — that, say the wise, is the highest state — the Kaivalaya Pad (the state of supreme realization).

It aims at samadhi (the final step in Patanjali's yoga system), whereby the individual is deindividualized and perceives within him the totality, unbounded and unembodied, limitless and free, all-pervading like the ether. It is seeing all things in the aspect of eternity.

A few words about the state of samadhi may not be amiss here. Samadhi may be conscious or super-conscious. In the one, the mind remains conscious of the object, while in the other, there is an inner calm in which one sees and gets a real insight, as if in a flash, of the object as it really is. It is seeing with the soul (or the inner spiritual eye), when our bodily eyes are shut. This is immediate and direct perceptual knowledge as distinct from mediate knowledge, i.e., through the medium of the smoke-colored glasses of the senses, the mind and the intellect. It is a state of "still silence," far removed from the maddening world outside. It is a mystical state in which chit, manas, budhi and ahankar all lose their respective functions and the disentangled and deindividualized Self alone shines in its own luminosity. It is about this state that Vyasa tells us: "Yoga can best be known only through yoga, for yoga becomes manifest through yoga." (Yoga Bhasya iii:6).

The most sacred syllable with the Raja yogins is Aum. In Mandukya Upanishad, we have a detailed account of this word. It is the same as the holy Word in the Gospel of St. John. It is the Kalma or Bang-i-Qadim of the Muslims, the Akash Bani or Vak Devi of the ancient Rishis, the Udgit or Naad of the Upanishads, the Sraosha of Zoroaster, and the

Naam or *Shabd* of the Masters. The world and the Vedas all originated from this syllable Aum. In Gita it is said, "The Brahmin, who reciting and thinking upon Aum, goes forth, abandoning the body, goes on to the highest path." Lord Krishna speaking of himself says, "I am *Omkar,* I am *Pranva* in all the Vedas, in speech I am *Ek-Akshra* (The One Syllable)." In the Upanishads it is stated, "Aum is the bow, the mind the arrow; Brahman is the target. Know ye the Brahman with concentration, hit the target with singleness of vision (*Ekagrat*), and then like an arrow becoming one with the target, the individual soul will become identified with the Brahman."

A single vibration in Brahman (*Eko Aham Bahusiam*) caused all the lokas, and with it brought into being all planes, spiritual, causal, astral and physical, with their countless divisions and subdivisions. The physical vibrations in man correspond to the one, original vibration that led to the projection of *Srishti* or the Universe, with all its trinities, like *Brahma, Vishnu* and *Siva; Satva, Rajas* and *Tamas; Jagrat, Swapan* and *Sushupti,* all of which are contained in Aum, the lord of the three worlds.

Lord Yama, the God of Death, exhorting Nachiketa said, "The goal uniformly extolled by all the Vedas, and for which man strives with all his tapas, is, in brief, Aum."

Similarly, the term *pranva* means something ever new and fresh, unchanging and eternal (*kutastha nitya*), like the relation between Shabda and its meaning, as opposed to *parinama nitya,* which is eternally changing.

From the above, it follows that each of the four classical forms of yoga is but an integral part of the yoga system as a whole as given by Patanjali, with a special emphasis on one or the other aspect of the system, and that these forms constitute a progressive development from Mantra Siddhi to Raja

Yoga, each step paving the way for the next higher stage on the yogic path.

To make yoga more practicable, distinctions were made in later times, for different types of people, based on individual temperaments and vocational pursuits. While the persons who were highly intellectual and reasoned out everything very often took to Jnana Yoga or "the Yoga of Knowledge," those with an emotional temperament were offered Bhakti Yoga or "the Yoga of Devotion," consisting of devotional exercises like singing and chanting of hymns and psalms (as did princess Mira and Chaitanya Mahaprabhu). Again, those who were primarily engaged in the outer activities of the world, were considered as best fitted for Karma Yoga or "the Yoga of Action," consisting of austerities like fasts and vigils, perform- ance of *yajnas* and other charitable acts, meritorious deeds like pilgrimages to holy places and reading of scriptures, etc., and above all the path of selfless duty. In this way there arose the three types of "popular yogas," namely those of head, heart and hand, signifying Jnana Yoga, Bhakti Yoga and Karma Yoga. These yogas find their first clear and unequivocal expo- sition in the Bhagavad Gita, and Lord Krishna stands in the same relationship to them as does Patanjali to the four tradi- tional types.

But it must be noticed that these three types cannot be classified into water-tight compartments. Each of them can hardly be practiced by itself to the total exclusion of the others. They simply indicate the predominant and inherent traits in the nature of the aspirants. A mere theoretical knowl- edge of yoga, without devotion and action, is just like a tree bereft of foliage and fruit, fit only for the woodcutter's axe. Again, devotion per se is meaningless, unless one has an intel- lectual grasp and a factual experience of the thing and actively strives for it. Actions by themselves, whether good or bad, without devotion and knowledge, keep one in perpetual bondage, like fetters of gold or of steel as the case may be, for both sorts have an equally binding force and efficacy. This world is a *Karma Kshetra,* or field of action, and all acts performed on the plane of the senses without discriminating knowledge and loving devotion bear fruit, which the doer has of necessity to gather up, whether he wills it or not. It is only action performed without attachment and desire for the fruit thereof that can bring freedom. One has therefore to become *Neh Karma* in this *Karma Bhoomi,* to escape from the wheel of Karmic bondage. The Law of Karma is stern and inexorable, and one should not unnecessarily go on doing Karmas endlessly and remain in eternal bondage.

He alone is free from the binding effect of Karmas,
who communes with the holy Word.

GURU AMAR DAS

The yoga system, thus, is in essence one integrated whole and cannot be split into any artifical classifications. In Bhagavad Gita or the Song Celestial, which pre-eminently is a Yoga Sutra, the prince of yogins, Lord Krishna, gives a clear exposition of the various types of yogas to the Kshatriya prince Arjuna, so as to bring home to him the importance of *Swadharm* or the Path of Duty, as defined from various angles, for work is nothing but worship, in the true sense of the word, if one realizes it as such and does it without attachment to the fruit thereof.

V. JNANA YOGA OR THE YOGA OF KNOWLEDGE
(RIGHT DISCRIMINATION)

The path of Jnana is for those who are gifted with strong intellect or mental grasp and have a keen insight, capable of penetrating into the why and wherefore of things, so as to reach the core of reality. It means right discrimination and knowledge, the very first essential in the eightfold path of

righteousness as enunciated by Buddha. It is from right understanding of the true values of life that everything else proceeds
in the right direction, for without right and correct knowledge
of Truth, all endeavors, with the best of intentions, are likely
to go awry and land us sooner or later into difficulties.

The importance of true knowledge is felt in fact in all
aspects of yogic life whether Karma Yoga or Bhakti Yoga. In
Karma Yoga, one needs to know and realize that one has a
right to action or work and not to the fruit thereof. As one
cannot but do work, the work is therefore to be performed in
the true spirit of one's duty, a dedication unto the Lord, with
the mind fixed on Him. The renunciation of attachment to
the fruits brings evenness of temper, and in the calm of self-
surrender lies true yoga of contemplation, a perfect peace born
of total surrender of one's life to God.

In Bhakti Yoga also, a bhakta or a devotee has, as a preliminary step, to understand the true significance of bhakti or
devotion to the Lord and then to develop in himself a correct
perspective, which may enable him to see the light of his *Isht-
Deva* not only in human beings but in every form of life.

In short, the path of Jnana Yoga lays emphasis on the true
knowledge of the inmost Reality that is, or the true nature of
atman. "Self-contemplation," the keynote of a true jnani, tries
with the exercise of proper discrimination, to separate the
apparently giant little self (the outer man) from the little
great Self within (the inner man), for the self is the foe of
Self, and self when properly trained becomes the friend of
Self. The aim of this yoga is to chase away the darkness of
ignorance with the torch of knowledge. It is a highly ana-
lytical path and for its successful working, one has to adhere
diligently to three things:

(i) *Shravan* or hearing: hearing the scriptures, the philosophic discourses, and above all, the living teachers of spirituality with first-hand experience of the Reality, who can trans-

mit their own life impulse to those coming into contact with them, for it is in the company of the truly awakened soul that one awakens from one's long slumber.

(ii) *Manan* or thinking: It consists in intense and thoughtful contemplation of what one has heard and understood so as to concretize the abstract, and make intellectual concepts the pulse of moment-to-moment living through a careful exercise of discrimination that distinguishes at every step the true from the false. It amounts to freeing the soul from the noose of egoism by all possible means at one's command. It is like churning butter out of the buttermilk.

(iii) *Nidhyasan* or practice: It consists in shifting the center of gravity from the ephemeral and changing self to the abiding and eternal Self, from the circumference to the center of one's being. This gradually brings about detachment from the pairs of opposites—riches and poverty, health and disease, fame and ignominy, pleasure and pain, etc.—into which one and all tend to drift in the normal course of existence.

The path of Jnana is a short-cut to yoga but it is frightfully steep, and very few can take to it. It requires a rare combination of razor-sharp intellect and intense spiritual longing, which only a few like Buddha and Shankara possess.

The path, however, would become smooth if one, by a mighty good fortune, were to meet a Master-soul. A Sant Satguru can, by his long and strong arm, draw an aspirant right out of the bottomless vortex of the life of the senses, without his having to do overmuch sadhna.

VI. BHAKTI YOGA OR THE YOGA OF LOVING DEVOTION

He who with unwavering devotion (Bhakti Yoga), does God service, has crossed beyond the strands, and is fit for salvation.

BHAGAVAD GITA

It is a yoga of worship with a loving and living faith, absolute and steadfast, in one's Isht-deva or the object of one's reverent adoration. It is a very popular path, most suited to those who are endowed with an emotional bent of mind. Selfless devotion is the keynote to success on this path. A bhakta or a devotee delights in rapturous strains, and is ever engaged in singing hymns in praise of his Lord and never gets weary of them. He tends to differ from a jnani both in his outlook on life and appioach to God, for instead of seeking the true Self, which is also the Brahman, he sets up a dualism between himself and his God, whom he adores as a separate and superior being. But this dualism is not necessarily ultimate; the bhakta knows the secret that one becomes that which one adores.

The cult of bhakti occupies an important integral place in all the yogic sadhnas. In a jnani, it provides substantial support in the form of devotion to the cause of self-knowledge. In a Karma yogin, it manifests itself in the form of an effect, and finds its efflorescence in acts of loving devotion for the common weal of all cieatures, for they are the creation of God.

The path of bhakti is characterized by three salient features: *japa*, *prem* and the symbolic representation of the object of veneration.

(i) *Japa*: It connotes the constant remembrance and repetition of God's name; in the beginning, orally, by means of the tongue, and then mentally. All the devotees engage in this practice irrespective of their religious orders. The practice of telling beads is widespread in the world. The Hindus name it *mala*, the Christians "rosary" and the Muslims *tasbih*. Unless it is performed with devotion and concentration, it defeats its purpose, for it runs the risk of becoming mechanical. Thus in some countries the whole practice has resolved itself into a mere rotating of a wheel on which are inscribed various prayers, only the hand being kept busy, while the mind instead of being fixed on God is left free to wander in worldly thoughts.

(ii) *Prem Bhava* or love-attitude assumes multitudinous forms with a bhakta. Sometimes, he assumes the role of a child, and clings to God as one does to his father or mother, and at other times altogether reverses the process and sports with Him as one does with his child. At times, he adopts an attitude of a friend and a companion (*sakha-bhava*), of a lover pining for his beloved spouse, of a devoted slave for his Master, or a tippler for the Saqi, as we find in the quatrains of Omar Khayyam. It all depends on one's varying moods and predilections. Christ always spoke of God as the "Father;" Paramhansa Ramakrishna adored Him as the "Mother;" Arjuna, the warrior prince, and Meera, the Rajput princess, always regarded Him as a *Sakha* or a friend and companion, while the Gopis sang songs of poignancy and grief as any love-smitten maiden would do for her lover.

(iii) Next comes the chosen symbol of the Lord. Everyone has his own conception of incarnations and God's manifesta-tions. As the Nameless assumes many names, so does the Formless appear in many forms according to the desires of His devotees. One may find Him in a stone as Sadna did, another in an idol, for He is immanent in all forms and answers to the prayers of all His sincere bhaktas and never lets them down. One can, of course, serve the Lord when He appears as a Godman, a teacher of humanity like Buddha, Christ, Kabir, Guru Nanak, who by their very presence illumine the world.

The process of bhakti gradually widens the outlook of a bhakta until he sees the light of his chosen idol pervading everywhere in and around him, and he begins to feel himself expanding with love, till he embraces the entire creation of God. This is the climax to which love brings him. The process was powerfully illustrated in our own time by the life of Sri Ramakrishna. At first he worshiped the Divine Mother as the idol in the Dakshineswar temple, then as the principle that manifested itself in all things good and holy, and finally, as the spirit that pervaded everything, the evil no less than the good, considering even the courtesan as its manifestation. The stages of the progress of a true bhakta from dualism to monism, from a limited individuality to universality, are traditionally termed as under:

(a) *Salokya*: The stage where the devotee desires to dwell in the same region as his Beloved.

(b) *Sampriya*: The stage where he not only wishes to dwell in the same region but also in close proximity to his Beloved.

(c) *Sarup*: The stage where the devotee wishes for himself the same form as that of his Beloved.

(d) *Sayuja*: The final stage when the devotee is content with nothing less than becoming one with the deity.

When a bhakta has reached the end of his journey, he no longer sees any duality, but beholds the one Deity pervading everything and everywhere. He may continue to speak of It in the manner in which he used to do, as a Father or a Mother, but he no longer knows any difference between that Being and himself, and so we read of Christ saying: "I and my Father are One."

VII. KARMA YOGA OR THE YOGA OF ACTION

Karma is the essence of existence, whether of man or of God, the Lord of Karma. Karmas rightly performed, in a spirit of service to the Divine, can lead to spiritual emancipation.

Karmas or actions are of two kinds: good and bad. Good deeds are those which tend to take us nearer to our spiritual goal while the bad deeds are those that take us farther away from it. There is no pleasure higher and more abiding than the one that comes from rediscovering one's true Self, which is really finding one's identity with the world around.

Life in all its forms is characterized by activity; and change is the law of life. No man can do without action, even for a fraction of a second. Wordsworth has described this state of perpetual activity thus:

> *The eye cannot choose but see,*
> *We cannot bid the ear be still,*
> *Our bodies feel where'er they be,*
> *Against or with our will.*

This being the case, what one has to do is to sublimate the course of one's actions, from end to end, so that they are purged of the dross of low and mean desires and sensual relationships. The selfless service of mankind is the highest virtue "Service before self" should then be the guiding principle in one's life. Since all life springs from God, the fountain of life and light, life must be made a perpetual dedication unto Him, without any desire for the fruit thereof. *Brahmsthiti* or establishment in Brahman comes not by renunciation of work (*saivyas*), but by giving up the desire for the fruits thereof (*tyaga*). It is not work, but the motive power behind the work, that binds us and pampers the ego.

Karma, to be the means of *moksha* or liberation from mind and matter, must satisfy three conditions:

(i) True knowledge of the higher values of life: Life itself being a continuous principle immanent in all forms of creation and is, therefore, worthy of respect and adoration. This is the realistic aspect of Karma.

(ii) Sincere and loving feelings toward all living creatures from the so-called lowest to the highest. This is the emotional aspect of Karma.

(iii) Karma must be performed with an active will, without fear of punishment or hope of reward. It should, in other words, be spontaneous, flowing automatically from one's spe-

cific nature (*swadharma*), i.e., from a sense of duty—work
for work's sake and not under any restraint or compulsion.
Man is not merely a creature of circumstances, but has a will
whereby he can modify his environment and direct his own
destiny. This is the volitional aspect of Karma.

A man who lives completely for others does not live for
himself, nor would he allow his ego to get inflated by thoughts
of possessiveness. With his spirit fully detached, a Karma yogin
lives in complete dissociation from his ordinary self.

> *He who does the task*
> *Dictated by duty,*
> *Caring nothing*
> *for the fruit of the action,*
> *He is a yogi.*
>
> BHAGAVAD GITA

In brief, "selfless devotion to duty" is the keynote to success
on the path of action. In the performance of duty, one must
rise above the sense-objects, the senses, the mind and the intelligent will, so that whatever is done from the fullness of one's
being will be a spontaneous act in the light of the atman, and
a righteous action; enabling one to see action in inaction and
inaction in action, and to be a still point in the ever-moving
wheel of life, which is at once in action and in inaction. In
this way, both the "action rightly performed" and "action
rightly renounced" lead to the same goal, for it is the right
understanding of the nature of action that brings the yogic
state.

These then are the three main types of yoga designed and
fashioned according to human nature. Each one receives the
mystic call, as one may be inclined temperamentally. To the
reflective philosopher gifted with a logical mind, it comes as
—"Leave all else and know me." The spiritual aspirant
endowed with an emotional mind gets it as—"Leave all else

and lose thyself in my love;" while a highly practical and active mind gets the call as—"Leave all else and serve me."

As has already been said, these three approaches tend to overlap and cannot be wholly separated. Something of the bhakta and the Karma yogin is present in the true jnani; something of the jnani and Karma yogin in the true bhakta; and something of the jnani and the bhakta in the true Karma yogin. The matter is not one of exclusiveness but of dominant tendency.

VIII. Other Yogas Mentioned in the Gita

Besides these well-known and popular forms, Lord Krishna gives us a few more types as well, with varying shades of distinction between them.

Yoga of Meditation

It is yoga of one-pointed attention, like the "light of a lamp in a windless place." It is for the self-controlled who can struggle hard. With the mind ever fixed on the atman, a person with the aid of an intelligent will gradually withdraws himself from the distractions of the mind, and finds himself a living and self-luminous soul and ever after moves toward perfection. For this, one has to divest himself of all aspirations, desires, hopes and possessions, and retire to a solitary place to practice control over mind and body.

Yoga of Spiritual Experience

This experience one gains by breaking through the three dimensional egg of gunas: satva, rajas and tamas, and by transcending the physical and mental states. It comes with the understanding of the true nature of things, i.e., vivek or discrimination. Its merit is greater than that of the performance of rites and rituals, sacrifices and ceremonials, scriptural studies and chantings of psalms, practice of austerities, and the giving of alms and doing of other charitable deeds, all of which are perforce done on and concerned with the plane of the senses, and cannot take one beyond.

Yoga of Mysticism

It is a refuge in the Lord by total self-surrender unto Him. It comes from knowledge of God's true nature and from direct vision. In this way, one frees himself from the good and evil effects of his actions, all of which he performs as an offering at the Lotus Feet of the Lord.

The Bhagavad Gita is truly a compendium of the yoga systems prevailing at the time of its exposition, and in fact mentions as many as eighteen: *Vikhad Yoga* (Ch. I), *Sankhya Yoga* (Ch. II), *Karma Yoga* (Ch. III), *Gyan-Karma-Sanyas Yoga* (Ch. IV), *Karma-Sanyas Yoga* (Ch. V), *Atam Sanjam Yoga* or *Dhyan Yoga* (Ch. VI), *Gyan-Vigyan Yoga* (Ch. VII), *Akshara-Brahma Yoga* (Ch. VIII), *Raja Vidya Raj Guhya Yoga* (Ch. IX), *Vibhuti Yoga* (Ch. X), *Vishva-Rup Darshan* (Ch. XI), *Bhakti Yoga* (Ch. XII), *Kshetra Kehetragya Vibhag Yoga* (Ch. XIII), *Gun Trai Vibhag Yoga* (Ch. XIV), *Purshottam Yoga* (Ch. XV), *Devasura Sampad Vibhag Yoga* (Ch. XVI), *Shradha Trai Vibhag Yoga* (Ch. XVII), and *Mokshar Sanyas Yoga* (Ch. XVIII).

From the above analysis, it is clear that the distinctions drawn between the various aspects of the yoga system are illustrative rather of the human mind's habit of looking at the same thing in different ways, then of any inherent difference between one type and another. They are just different facets of the same subject, and they often overlap and interpenetrate each other. If one studies the Gita closely enough, one will begin to see that while Lord Krishna speaks of different yogas to harmonize with varying human approaches to the Divine, the practical esoteric discipline that accompanies them is the same. When he initiated Arjuna into the mystic science, he opened his *Divya Chakshu* or third eye, and it was only subsequently that the prince could behold him in his Universal Form or *Vishva Roopa* (Ch. XI). Finally, as Guru, the great royal yogi told him to leave all else and surrender himself completely to him; *Sarva Dharman parityajya mam ekam sharanam vraja* (Ch. XVIII). Further hints of the inner path are not lacking in the Gita; thus in Chapter I, we are told that at the very outset the Lord sounded the five-melodied conch. But in the absence of a teacher who has himself practically mastered the science, we tend to treat it either on the level of intellectual discussion or that of ritual chanting, thus missing its inner import.

It may be noted that the dualistic assumption characterizes the first stages not only of Bhakti Yoga, but of all the other types of yoga as well. They begin by distinguishing the jiva from the Brahman; one imperfect, finite and limited, and the other Perfect, Infinite and Limitless. Creation itself is the product of two principles, the positive and the negative: *Sat* and *Sato* in the purely spiritual world, *Purush* and *Prakriti* at the higher reaches of Brahmand, *Brahma* and *Shakti* in mid-Brahmand, *Kal* and *Maya* still lower and *Jyoti* and *Niranjan* at the bottom of the Brahmand. It is the union of these, whatever the stage, that brings the various forms into manifestation, from the minutest atom to the largest Universe. The term *Brahman* itself comes from two roots: *vireh* which denotes growth or expansion, and *manan* which connotes cognition. The process of creation is one in which the Unity projects itself into dualistic and pluralistic forms, and the way back is through the reverse process from duality and plurality to Unity. But so long as a person remains in the body, he cannot, according to the yogins, be always in a state of samadhi or union with the Adi Purush, the Primal Being. The yoga system therefore believes in *vedeh mukti,* or final liberation only after death. Again, the highest heaven of the yogins is Sahasrar, the region of the thousand-petaled lights, and that of the Yogishwars is Trikuti, the headquarters of the Brahmand, the origin or the egg of Brahman itself. Most of the Prophets of the world descend from this region, which is a half-way house between the physical and the purely spiritual realms, and at times refer to the beyond as Par Brahm only. The path of the Saints and the Masters, however, goes beyond these, for they speak definitely of Sat Lok, the abode of the True One, the realm of pure spirit, and of regions even beyond thereto: Alakh, Agam and Anami.

IX. Yoga in the Zoroastrian Scriptures

It will be of interest to know that we have, in the Gathas of Zoroaster, a five-fold system of the Beatific Union with Ahura Mazda, which corresponds closely to the yogic systems like Jnana, Bhakti, Karma, Raja Yoga, etc., that we have been examining. We quote in extenso from *Practical Metaphysics of Zoroastrians* by Mr. Minochehr Hormusji Toot, a leading Zoroastrian scholar.

(i) *Gatha Ahura Vaiti* — The Path of Divine Knowledge:

Look within with the penetrating enlightened mind and search out the truth for your personal self so as to overpower the base self and gross physical selfish egoism, *akeen,* by the evolution of the better and higher self, *vahyo,* and ultimately to realize the best, Absolute Being (*Vahisht Ahura*), and the highest self, of Ahura Mazda or the Ultimate Reality of the Universe, *Asha Vahishta.*

The polarity of the "Better and the Base," the primordial, spiritual subtlety and the grossest inertia, is created by the twin spirit forces: the unfolding (*spento*) and the straightening (*angoo*), produced by Mazda. Both the Life and the

Matter produced by the harmonious coalescence of these twin spirit forces, evolve toward perfection by their related activity.

The above is the metaphysical path of spiritual knowledge, as given by the Gatha Ahura Vaiti (Refer Jnana Yoga).

(ii) *Gatha Ushta Vaiti* — the Path of Love and Devotion:

The Path of *Armaiti,* Divine Love and Devotion, acquired by steadfast attachment to the Truthful Beloved Master Ratu Zarathustra. Considering the Beloved Master, connected with the All-pervading, Infinite Reality, as all in all, the alpha and the omega, the devotee remains detached from and unentangled with worldly attachments, and procures the divine love, which seeks and cherishes the Beatific Union with the All-pervading Reality after Creator Ahura Mazda.

Thus proclaims Ratu Zarathustra in this Gatha:

> *Thus I reveal the Word, which the most Unfolded*
> *One has taught me,*
> *The Word which is the Best for the mortals to listen;*
> *Whosoever shall render obedience and steadfast*
> *attention unto me, will attain for one's own self,*
> *the All embracing Whole Being and Immortality;*
> *And through the service of the Holy Divine Spirit*
> *will realize Mazda Ahura.*
>
> (Ha. 45-8 — Refer Bhakti Yoga)

(iii) *Gatha Spenta Mainyu* — the Path of Selfless Service:

> *Selfless service is rendered for the furtherance,*
> *growth and benevolence of the entire Universe and*
> *all living beings therein:*
> *The Unitive Knowledge is best for men since their*
> *birth,*
> *Let the selfless service be rendered for the Universe,*
> *This Universe must prosper for our sublimation.*
>
> (Ha. 8:5)

We must sacrifice the finite self, ego or individuality at the altar of benevolent, philanthropic service of the entire Universe, in order to acquire the Infinite vision of the Unity of Life and the immanence of the All-pervading Reality through the worship of Ahura Mazda, the Creator, Source, and Ultimate Goal of all.

The Gatha ends with the soul-strirring axiom of life:

> *The Most-Sublimating, Ennobling Will or Volition is that of righteous service.*
> *Which the Creator of the individualized human existence culminates with the Enlightened Super Mind.*

(Refer Karma Yoga)

(iv) *Gatha Vahu — Khshetra* or the Path of Self-Mastery:

By controlling the base mental propensities and mean tendencies of physical nature, through the sublimation of the volition power, aspiring to the Divine Kingdom of the communion of the All-loving and All-pervading Ahura Mazda, the self-mastery is attained with calm and composed mind.

The Holy Self-mastery is the most sustaining absolute sovereignty.
By introspecting worshipful service, it is procured inwardly through the All-pervading Reality,
O Mazda! Let us achieve that best now.

(Ha. 51:1—Refer Raja Yoga)

(v) Next we have the Gatha of *Vahishto Ishtish,* which deals with the Path of self-sublimation. It consists in physical, mental and spiritual culture by cultivation of higher and nobler qualities of head and heart, in trying to realize one's true self in relation to the Highest Self of Ahura Mazda, and in dedicating the finite self and relative being to Ahura Mazda.

The life on earth is a great sacrifice, *Yajna* (yagna)—the voluntary sacrifice of self for the well-being of one's fellow beings.

It is in self-sublimation that all human endeavors ultimately end, and in fact, it is the objective to which all the paths as described above lead. Without true knowledge of the twin spirit forces, the better and the base, loving devotion of the aspirant to the great cause, and selfless service, one cannot master the self-assertive self within him so as to rise above body-consciousness, and thus prepare himself for the spiritual path that lies ahead.

In Zoroastrian philosophy, the twin principles, or the "Better and Base spirit forces," is the fundamental law of the relative existence manifested in the Universe. This polarity is essential for the evolution of life, from the grossest base to the better and higher stages of spirituality, right up to realizing the infinite goodness and supreme benevolence of the Absolute Being beyond them. Without this polarity of the Better and the Base, the best of the Absolute Beyond can never be realized and the Impersonal Supreme Being cannot be comprehended:

> *Indeed unto one's self as the best of all,*
> *The Self-Radiant person shall impart Self-Enlight-*
> *   enment,*
> *So that, O Omniscient Mazda, thou shalt reveal*
> *   Thyself,*
> *Through Thy Most Benevolent spirit, and shall*
> *   grant*
> *The Blissful Wisdom of the Divine Mind,*
> *Through the All-pervading Reality.*
>
> GATHA USHTAVAITI

In the Venidad, the Supreme Ahura Mazda assures us, thus:

> *Indeed I shall not allow the Twin opposite spirit forms to stand in contest against the superman who is advancing toward the Best Absolute Being.*
> *The stars, moon and sun, O Zarathustra, praise such a person;*
> *I praise him, I the Creator Ahura Mazda,*
> *Hail of Beatitude unto thee,*
> *O Superman! Thou who hast come from the perishable place to the Imperishable.*

VENIDAD

X. YOGA AND THE OUTER SCIENCES

Having discussed in some detail the various methods of yoga, we may in conclusion, remind ourselves of the true warning sounded by Shankara:

> The three-fold path; the path of the world, the path of desires, and the path of scriptures, far from giving the knowledge of Reality, keeps one perpetually bound in the prison-house of the Universe. Deliverance comes only when one frees himself from this iron chain.
>
> Liberation cannot be achieved except by the perception of the identity of the individual spirit with the Universal spirit. It can be achieved neither by yoga, nor by Sankhya, nor by the practice of religious ceremonies, nor by mere learning.

SHANKARACHARYA

To bring up to date Shankara's message that True Knowledge is a matter of direct perception and not mere ceremony, ritual or inference, we may add that it cannot come through the outer sciences either. The discoveries of the modern physical sciences have indeed been spectacular, and have confirmed many of the views about the nature of the cosmos and of existence voiced by the yogic systems. They have established, beyond doubt, that everything in the universe is relative, and that all forms are fundamentally brought into existence by the interplay of positive and negative energies. These discoveries have led some to presume that physical sciences can and will lead us to the same knowledge that yogins in the past sought through yoga; that science will replace yoga and make it irrelevant.

A blind man, though he may not be able to see the sun, may yet feel its heat and warmth. His awareness of some phenomenon which he cannot directly perceive, may lead him to devise and perform a series of experiments in order to know its nature. These experiments may yield him a lot of valuable data. He may be able to chart more accurately, perhaps, than the normal man, the course of the sun, its seasonal changes and the varying intensity of its radiation. But can all this knowledge that he has gathered be a substitute for a single moment's opportunity to view the sun directly for himself?

As with the blind man and the man of normal vision, so too with the scientist and the yogin. The physical sciences may yield us a lot of valuable, indirect knowledge of the Universe and its nature, but this knowledge can never take the place of direct perception, for just as the blind man's inferential knowledge cannot get at the sun's chief attribute which is light, so too the scientist in his laboratory cannot get at the cosmic energy's chief attribute, which is Consciousness. He may know a great deal about the universe, but his knowledge can never add up to universal consciousness. This consciousness can only be attained through the inner science, the science of yoga, which by opening our inner eye, brings us face to face with the Cosmic Reality. He whose inner eye has been opened, no longer needs to rely on spiritual hearsay, the assertions of his teacher, or mere philosophic or scientific inference.

He sees God for himself and that exceeds all proof. He can
say with Christ, "Behold the Lord!" or with Guru Nanak,
"The Lord of Nanak is visible everywhere," or with Sri
Ramakrishna, "I see Him just as I see you—only very much
more intensely" (when replying to Naren—as Vivekananda
was then known—on his very first visit, in answer to his
question: "Master, have you seen God?").

CHAPTER FOUR

Advaitism

Y OGA is as timeless as Brahman Itself. As with every fresh
cycle man comes to an awareness of the All-pervading, he
tries to discover the means for realizing It. It was Hiranyagarbha, we are told, who first taught yoga or the Divine Way,
but it was his successors, Gaudapada and Patanjali, who
developed it into a regular system. As we have already seen
in the foregoing chapter, all true yoga begins with a dualistic
assumption but ends in a non-dualistic one. It is not surprising, therefore, that many students of the inner science should
have been confounded by this paradox. As time passed, confusion led to controversy, and a half-truth was often mistaken
for the full truth. It was at such a time that Shankara, the
prodigy from South India, arose to preach the true philosophy
of Advaitism.

He was gifted with amazing powers of reasoning, logic and
insight and few have attained to the depth, sublety and con-
sistency of vision that are to be found in Shankara's writings.
Taking up all the great scriptures as they came down from
the past, he unequivocally interpreted their meaning and
established their identity of substance. He showed that the
Reality was One and, in its ultimate analysis, could not tol-
erate any pluralism or dualism. An individual jiva might
begin as distinct from the Brahman, but by the time he had
attained full realization, he would have realized his oneness
with the Absolute, the All-pervading. Armed with clairvoyant
intellectual power, he swept Indian thought clean of all the

seeming contradictions that were clogging its free development.

We may now examine some of the basic concepts that he taught.

Self — the basis of conscious life

Shankara regarded the empirical life of the individual consciousness as nothing but a waking dream, and as any other dream, an unreal substance. Its unreality comes to light when one travels from limited to cosmic consciousness, or contemplates the relative nature of physical consciousness as it varies from waking (*jagrat*), to dream (*swapan*), and from dream to dreamlessness (*sushupti*). If empirical experience is relative in character, wherein lies its reality? The answer provided by Shankara is that it is to be sought in the Thinking Mind, which in turn only reflects the light of the Atman, the Eternal Self, the unchanging, the absolute, the real witness (*sakshi*).

The principle of causality is just a condition of knowledge. The objects appear to be real so long as we work within the limits of cause and effect. The moment we rise above these limitations, all objects vanish into airy nothings. In the true nature of reality, there is no place for causation, because causal explanations are always incomplete and ultimately lead nowhere. The objects momentarily appear as bubbles or ripples on the surface of the water and disappear the next moment into the water and are no more. Water alone remains the real substratum of the whole phenomenon. In just the same way, the Real contains and transcends the phenomenal, and is free from all relationships of time, space and cause. The entire world lives in the mind of man, and it is the movement of the conscious mind that produces the distinctions of perception, the perceiver and the perceived, a differentiation where in fact there is none, as everything is part of the vast ocean of unity. This state does not recognize the distinctions of knower, known and knowledge, all of which are but relative terms with no finality about them. Similarly, the three states of the human experience (waking, dreaming and the dreamless) are unreal, for none of them lasts long enough, and each gives place to the other in turn, as the mind passes from state to state. Each of them has a beginning and an end and exists only in the absence of the others. The term "relativity" in itself implies its antithesis, the "Reality," and beyond the three states specified above lies the atman, as the basis of them all. It alone is and constantly remains, behind the ever changing panorama of life, the ever unborn, eternally awake, the dreamless and self-illumined, by its very nature a pure cognition distinct from the non-cognition of the sleep state.

The nature of creation

Creation as such does not exist per se. The actual and the real is ever the same and is not subject to change. The unconditioned cannot be conditioned as infinity cannot be finitized. All that is, is Brahman, and there can be nothing apart from the Absolute Unity. It projects Itself into varying forms, which are an expression of Its power; but if we perceive them in terms of plurality or duality and of limitation, it is not that such qualities inhere in the Absolute, but that our own perception is limited by the narrow, everyday, human consciousness. He who has passed from *avidya* to *vidya,* from ignorance to knowledge, knows the world of the relative to be only *maya* or illusion, and sees the Absolute in everything, just as he who knows the true nature of ice sees it only as another form of water. The power of the Absolute, popularly known as Ishwar and called the Creator, is the root-cause of all consciousness. The world of plurality or duality is mere *maya* (an instrument for measuring things on the level of the intellect), while the real One is non-dual and hence is at once measureless and immeasurable. To use the well-known simile—"The variety subsists in the atman, as does a snake in the rope or a ghost in the stump of a tree." As an empirical experience is neither identical with the atman, nor exists apart from or independent of the atman, so the world is neither one with the atmán nor separate from it.

Atman is one and universal, unconditioned and limitless like space, but when conditioned by mind and matter, it looks like *Ghat-Akash* or space enclosed in a pitcher, yet becomes one with the universal space when the pitcher breaks apart. All the differences, then, are but in name, capacity and form. The jiva and the atman are one and of the same essence. Kabir, speaking of it, says that the spirit is part and parcel of Ram, or the All-pervading Power of God. The Muslim divines also describe it (*rooh*) as *Amar-i-Rabbi*, or the fiat of God. While the jiva is conditioned and limited by the limiting adjuncts, physical, mental and causal, the atman or the disembodied jiva, freed from these finitizing adjuncts, is limitless and unconditioned.

The Self or Atman

The basis of truth lies in Self-certainty. The Self precedes everything else in the world. It comes even before the stream of consciousness and all concepts of truth and untruth, reality and unreality, and before all considerations, physical, moral and metaphysical. Consciousness, knowledge, wisdom and understanding presuppose some kind of energy known as "Self" to which all these are subservient; and in fact, they flow from it. All physical and mental faculties, even the vital airs and empirical experiences, appear in the light of the shining Self, the self-illuminated atman. They all have a purpose and an end that lie far deeper than themselves and which form the springboard for all kinds of activity, whether physical, mental and supramental. All these, however, fail to grasp the real nature of the Self, being themselves in a state of continuous flux. Self being the basis of all proof and existing before proof, cannot be proved. How can the Knower be known, and by whom? Self is in fact, the essential nature of everyone, even that of the atheist. This Self then, is eternal, immutable and complete, and in its essence, is ever the same at all times, under all conditions and in all states.

The nature of Self

Though we know that the Self exists, yet we do not know what it is, for knowledge itself follows the Self and is due to and because of the Self. The true nature of the Self may however be comprehended by the Self, if It could be stripped of all the enshrouding sheaths of senses, mind, understanding and will, in which it is clothed and covered. What is then left is variously described as "Undifferentiated Consciousness," "Eternal Knowledge" or "Pure Awareness," and is characterized by the Light of the Great Void. It is the supreme principle whose essential nature is self-effulgence. It is infinite, transcendental and the essence of absolute knowledge. It has three attributes of *Sat, Chit* and *Anand,* i.e., pure existence, pure knowledge and pure bliss. As the Self is complete in Itself, and by Itself, It has no activity of Its own, nor has any need for it, nor requires any outside agency. All-pervading and self-existent, It knows no limits and no motives.

Individual knowledge and consciousness

Though the ultimate reality is the non-dual spirit, yet determinate knowledge and empirical experience presuppose the existence of: (i) The knower, or the subject that knows apart from the internal organ behind the senses and the object known. The knowing mind is but a reflecting mirror that reflects the luminosity of the atman, in which knowledge grows. (ii) The process of knowledge as determined by modifications in the internal organ: *vritis* or undulations creating ripples and bubbles in the stream of consciousness. These vritis are of four kinds: the Indeterminate (*manas* or the mindstuff), the Determinate (*budhi* or intelligent will), Self-sense (*ahankar* or the self-assertive ego), and the Subconscious (*chit* or the deep and hidden potencies). (iii) The object known through the light of the atman as reflected by the internal organ (*antahkaran*).

Knowledge and its sources

Knowledge is of two kinds; ultimate and final, or empirical and relative. Knowledge in its ultimate reality is a state of being and never grows. It is already there and is revealed by the light of the atman, which transcends at once both the subject apprehending and the object apprehended, beyond which there is nothing.

True knowledge is purely an action of the soul and is perfect in itself and independent of the senses and the sense organs. "An all-knowing mind," says Professor J. M. Murray, "embraces the totality of being under the aspect of eternity. As we gain our entrance into the world of being, a total vision is ours." According to Shankara, "highest knowledge is the immediate witness of reality itself," for then, the knower and the known become one reality. But the real Self which is pure awareness cannot be the object of knowledge.

The empirical knowledge of the external world is just like animal knowledge. It is based on and derived from the sense organs, and as such has forms and modes all of which are conspicuous by their absence from true knowledge. But nothing becomes real till it is experienced. Even a proverb is no proverb until it is illustrated in actual life and practice.

All empirical knowledge is revealed either by perception or by scriptural testimony. The human perception has never been considered true, perfect and accurate. One may see a snake in a rope, or a ghost in the stump of a tree. Generally, things are not what they seem to be. The colors of things we see are those that are not absorbed by them, but are rejected and thrown out. The redness of the rose is not part of the rose but something alien to it. Again, inference and scriptural testimony are not altogether infallible. The source of inference is previous experience, which is itself fallible and even if it were not, situations in the present may not wholly fit in with the knowledge gained in the past. This is the case even with intuition, which is the sum-total of all experience in the subconscious. A cloud of smoke on the top of a distant hill may be indicative of fire or it may be a sheet of fog. Similarly, scriptural testimony, though admitted as an infallible and certain source of knowledge, cannot always be treated as such. The Vedas, which constitute the Divine knowledge, appear and disappear with the rise and dissolution of each cycle of time. They are supposed to be an inexhaustible mine of universal and ideal knowledge. But the term "knowledge" implies a record of spiritual experiences gained at the supersensory planes. The moment the experiences thus gained are translated into human language and reduced to writing, they acquire form and method, and the moment they acquire form and method, they lose their freshness and life, their quality of limitless being. That which cannot be limited or defined, begins to be treated as something defined and limited, and instead of the scriptures giving vital knowledge, they tend to distract men from it by offering only abstractions. At best they can only point toward the Truth, but they can never give it. The concepts of the Universal as contained therein, remain as mere concepts, for they can neither be received, inferred nor correctly communicated; they begin to have meaning only when one learns to rise above the empirical plane and experiences Truth for himself.

From the above, one comes to the irresistible conclusion that "seeing," or direct and immediate perception, is above all proof and testimony. It is seeing in the pure light of the atman, which is free from even the least shadow of correlativity. It is nothing but a direct, integral experience of the soul. *Sruti*, or revealed scripture, without first-hand inner experience, is sound without sense. All flights of thought, imagination or fancy, and all empirical knowledge, are inadequate and cannot do justice to Truth or the Ultimate Reality. *Anubhava* is verily the real and absolute knowledge, and is knowledge of the Absolute. It is the self-certifying experience of the soul, which bears testimony to the recorded spiritual experience of the sages as given in the srutis.

The nature of Brahman

The very idea of finitude implies the existence of the Infinite, as does the word "unreal" of something real, the basis of all intelligence and imagination. Again, we have the overwhelming testimony of scriptural texts, which speak of religious experiences of all seers at all times and in all places.

The nature of Brahman cannot be expressed in words. It is the foundation of all that exists. It spreads everywhere, and at the same time is nowhere in relation to anything particular. It is a paradox at once of being and non-being. There are two ways of looking at the problem: the negative way and the positive way. There is God, the Incomprehensible Absolute, and God Who actually creates, works, and is the First Cause, and is known variously as the *Logos* or the Holy Spirit, the *Kalma* or the *Bang-i-Qadim*, the *Naad* or the *Udgit*, the *Naam* or the *Shabd*. The latter terms indicate the life-principle, the Word or the Power of God that is immanent and vibrates everywhere from the highest to the lowest in the Universe. It is both the material and the efficient cause of the world. It is the principle of Truth and the spirit of God (God-in-action—*Ekankar*). Of this Power of God, the Gospels tell us that, "The Light shineth in darkness and the darkness comprehendeth it not." This power of Brahman (Ishvara) or Godhead is the medium between Brahman and the Universe and partakes of the nature of both. But His oneness is not affected by self-expression into many—*Eko aham bahusiam.* The two exist as reality and appearance, and the difference arises because of the limited insight in man.

To sum up, the Supreme Reality is the basis of the world as we know it, speak of it and see it. The plurality, or diversity in unity, is the result of erroneous judgment. The world is unreal but not a subjective illusion. The Absolute is in the world but the world is not the Absolute, for a shadow cannot take the place of the substance. A thing based on the real cannot be the "real" itself. The world is but the phenomenal truth and not the essential truth of the Reality, or the centripetal force at the core of it.

The individual self is a complexity of likes and dislikes, preferences and prejudices, purposes and projects, memories and associations. The conditioned jiva is essentially the unconditioned atman. This empirical self or the individual understanding is, through ignorance of its own real nature, the active doer, the enjoyer and the sufferer in the pure light of the atman, of which it has no knowledge nor any experience. Enclosed in the physical body, composed of five elements (ether, air, fire, water and earth), is the subtle body consisting of seventeen elements (five organs of perception: eyes, ears, nose, tongue and skin; five of action: sight, hearing, smell, taste and touch; the five vital airs, and manas and budhi), and also the causal or seed body. The self follows the inexorable law of karma as it migrates from one body to another on the giant Wheel of Life. These limiting adjuncts (the physical, mental and causal), reduce the atman to the level of a jiva (individual consciousness), and determine its fate, taking it into endless gyres. In the core of the jiva is the

Witnessing Self, that merely looks on and sheds luster on the entire stage and, while illumining the ego, mind, senses and the sense objects, continues to shine in Its own light, even when the stage is cleared. It is against this illumined silver screen that the whole show takes place.

The attainment of the state where the atman knows itself for what it is and realizes that it is naught but Brahman, is the goal of Advaitism. This state is one of direct experience and, as Shankara has made abundantly clear, it cannot be attained merely by ratiocination, the reading of scriptures or the performance of rituals. It can come only through the pursuit of yoga, and the essential thing to be remembered is that Advaitism by itself is not a yoga but, strictly speaking, represents the philosophy of yoga at its subtlest and profoundest. Shankara, as he himself clarified, was not speaking of something new. He was engaged in the task of reformulating what had already been expressed in the Upanishads and the Gita. Endowed with an extraordinary intellect and an amazing flair for logic, he set about restating in a coherent and systematic form the insight embedded in the srutis, which in subsequent times had been confused and had led to much needless controversy. He demonstrated once and for all that any approach to Brahman which did not preach the non-pluralistic and non-dualistic reality was in its very nature illogical, and that Advaitism was in fact the logical conclusion of yogic thought. Implicit in this approach was the view that of all states of samadhi, the one in which the individual atman lost its identity in the Brahman (called *Nirvikalp Samadhi*), was the highest. This state was to be attained here and now, and one could be free in this life (*jivan mukta*). He who had plumbed beneath the phenomenal to the Absolute, would never again be taken in by appearances. He was a liberated spirit, living in the light of True Knowledge. Past actions might carry him onward through physical existence, but once these were exhausted, he was absorbed wholly into the Brahman, the pure cognition.

Shankara was indeed a remarkable man of learning and insight and his contribution to Indian thought is permanent. In carrying it to its logical conclusion, he gave it the brilliance of consistent clarity. But just as ritual and scripture cannot be a substitute for direct inner experience, likewise merely knowing that the Self and the Brahman are One cannot take the place of an actual experience of this union. The philosophy of yoga is not the same thing as yoga. At best, it can only clear our thinking of its present confusion and point out the final goal to be attained, but the rest must remain a matter of practical and personal realization through yoga.

PART TWO

The Study of Surat Shabd Yoga

CHAPTER FIVE

Surat Shabd Yoga

The Yoga of the Celestial Sound Current

I N THE foregoing sections of this study, we have seen how it has been taught since time immemorial by the Indian sages that behind the apparent self of which we are conscious in everyday existence, the self that shirks pain and seeks pleasure, that changes from moment to moment and is subject to the effect of time and space, there is the permanent "Self," the Atman. This Atman forms the basic reality, the final substance, the essence of essences, and it is in the light of its being that all else assumes meaning. Likewise, we have seen how the Indian mystics have analysed the nature of the Universe. Seen from the surface, our world appears to be a queer composition of contradictory elements. Faced with these contradictions, man is compelled to look for a Creator who holds the opposing forces in balance and represents permanence behind the flux of existence. But as he penetrates deeper and still deeper, he discovers that the contradictions are only apparent, not real: that far from being opposed in nature, they are differentiated manifestations of the same Power, and that they are not even "manifestations" properly so called, but are illusions of the ignorant mind which are dispelled in the light of realization when one begins to know that the ocean is changeless though it appears to change.

These two insights are basic to Indian thought, and on closer examination will be seen to be not separate, but one.

The recognition of the absolute nature of the inner Self, the Atman, implies recognition of the true nature of existence of the Paramatman, the Brahman; while an understanding of the nature of Paramatman or Brahman implies an understanding of the Atman. If behind the changing, time-ridden self, there be an eternal, changeless and timeless One, and if behind the flux of mutability of the creation as we normally know it, there be an Absolute Immutable Reality, then the two must be related and must in fact be identified. How can there be two Absolutes? How can the Atman be distinct from the Brahman, when all that is, is only a projection of Brahman?

The moment we realize these truths about the nature of Self and Overself, or the One Truth about the nature of Reality, the problem that inevitably poses itself is: Why do we in everyday existence experience the world in terms of duality and plurality, feeling ourselves separate from each other and from life in general, and what may be the means for transcending this unnecessary constriction of ourselves and merging into the Ocean of Consciousness that is our essential state? The answer to the first part of this question has been that the spirit, in its downward descent, gets enveloped in fold upon fold of mental and material apparatus which compel it to experience life in terms of their limitations, until, no longer conscious of its own inherent nature, the soul identifies itself with their realm of time and space — *nam-rup-prapanch*. The answer to the second part has been that the soul can bear witness to itself, provided it can divest itself of its limiting adjuncts. The many forms and variations of yoga that we have examined are no more than the various methods evolved for accomplishing this process of disentanglement or spiritual involution.

The one recurring theme in the teachings of all great rishis and mystics has been that their insights are based not on inherited learning, philosophical speculation or logical reasoning, but on first-hand inner experience or *anubhava*—a word whose lucidity of expressiveness defies translation. They explain that seeming differences are not because of any contradiction inherent in what they say, but because men vary greatly in temperament, and what is possible for the man of a cultured and refined intelligence is impossible for the unsophisticated peasant, and vice versa. Various rivers may wend through different plains, but they all reach the sea. Patanjali's Eightfold Path is the first major attempt to correlate the many available avenues into a single coherent system for spiritual reintegration. Later rishis and teachers derived much guidance from him, but their teachings implicitly embody the recognition that his system is too exacting and tends to deny spiritual attainment to the average man. Furthermore, it is so complex that for the majority of *sadhaks* (aspirants) it is likely to become a maze in which they lose their way and mistake the intermediate goals for the final destination. And so, while Mantra Yoga, Laya Yoga, Hatha Yoga and especially Raja Yoga carry on Patanjali's tradition in modified forms, there emerge three other major forms that represent, in contrast to the Ashtanga Marg, a great simplification and specialization. The Jnana yogin, the Karma yogin or the bhakta no longer needs to retire from the world or undergo exacting psycho-physical disciplines. Each approaches the goal from a particular angle and reaches it by sheer purposeful concentration.

The end of all yoga, as Shankara clarified, is absorption into the Brahman. All the paths therefore aim at samadhi, in which state such experience can be attained. But if Patanjali's system and its derivatives have certain serious drawbacks, it is a question whether the three other major forms are wholly without them. If for the Karma yogin freedom lies through detachment and desirelessness, is it possible for him to be completely free? Does he not seek emancipation in following his path, and is not that itself a form of desire? Besides, is it psychologically possible for the human mind to detach itself completely from its normal field of experience without first anchoring itself in another and higher one? It is a universal characteristic of man that he seeks kinship with something other than himself. This is the law of his life and source of all his great achievements. The child is bound to his toys, and the adult to family and society. As in the case of a child, you may not without harm deprive him of his playthings until he has outgrown them psychologically, likewise to expect the sadhak to give up his social and family attachments without first outgrowing them by discovering something greater and larger, is to cut at the root of life. It will not bring progress but regression, for the man who undertakes it as an enforced discipline only succeeds in repressing his natural desires. The result is not the enhancement of consciousness but its numbing and atrophy, not detachment but indifference. This, as Mr. T. S. Eliot has pointed out, "differed completely" from both "attachment" and "detachment," resembling

> ... the others as death resembles life, being between two lives — unflowering, between the live and the dead nettle.

The discipline of Karma Yoga is a necessary one, but if it is to fulfill its end it must be completed by another discipline of an esoteric kind, without which it tends to reduce itself to an ineffectual attempt to lift oneself up by one's shoestrings.

As for the Jnana yogin, jnana may carry him very far indeed. It may take him beyond the gross physical plane into the spiritual ones. But can jnana carry him beyond itself? And if jnana, which as we have seen, forms one of the koshas that encompass the atman, albeit a very rarefied one, how can it then give the soul absolute freedom? Jnana is the help and yet it may prove to be the hindrance. It has indubitably the power to rid the soul of all encumbrances grosser than itself, but having reached thus far it tends to clog further progress. And since it is not of the true essence of the soul, the Absolute, it cannot be wholly above the reach of *Kala* or Time. Mystics distinguish between the two realms of time, *Kala* and *Mahakala*, thus: the first of these extends over the physical world and the less gross regions immediately above it, whereas the second stretches to all the higher planes that are not of pure spirit. Hence, the gains that the jnani achieves may be out of the reach of time as we normally conceive it (*kala*), but they are not wholly beyond the reach of greater time (*mahakala*). It need hardly be pointed out that what is true of Jnana Yoga is also true of those forms of yoga that depend upon the pranic energies. They too are not of the true nature of the Atman, and as such cannot lead It to a state of Absolute Purity, beyond the realm of relativity.

Besides its inability to ensure absolute freedom, Jnana Yoga is not a path accessible to the average man. It demands extraordinary intellectual powers and stamina which few possess. It was to meet this difficulty as well as that posed by Karma Yoga when practiced by itself, that Bhakti Yoga came into prominence. He who normally would not be able to detach himself from the world nor had the mental powers to analyse the true Self from the untrue could by the power of love leap or bridge the gap and reach the goal. But how can man love that which has neither form nor shape? So the bhakta anchors himself in the love of some *Isht-deva*, some definite manifestation of God. But in overcoming this practical difficulty he exposes himself to the same limitations as the jnani. The chosen Isht-deva by its very nature represents a limitation upon the Nameless and Formless Absolute. And even if the bhakta reaches the level of that manifestation, can that limited being take him beyond itself to that which has no limitation?

A study of the lives of the prominent exponents of this system clarifies the point. Ramanuja, the well-known mystic of the Middle Ages, failed to apprehend the teachings of his predecessor, Shankara. He followed what in Indian philosophy is known as the school of *vasisht advaita,* i.e., that the Atman can reach Ishwar (God as the manifested Creator of the Universe), and can get saturated with cosmic consciousness, but it can never become one with Him. What to say then of reaching God as the Unmanifested, Nameless Brahman? The experience of Sri Ramakrishna in our own time once again brings out this limitation. He had always been a worshiper of the Divine Mother and she often blessed him with her visions. But he always perceived her as something other than himself, as a power outside himself and one for whose operation he could often become a medium, but in which he could not merge himself. When he subsequently met Totapuri, an advaita sanyasin, he realised that he must get beyond this stage to one where there was no name or form and where the Self and the Overself became one. When he attempted to enter into such a state he discovered that his earlier attainments became a hurdle in spite of all his efforts. He tells us:

I could not cross the realm of name and form and bring my mind to the unconditioned state. I had no difficulty in withdrawing my mind from all objects except one, and this was the all too familiar form of the Blissful Mother — radiant and of the essence of pure consciousness — which appeared before me as a living reality and would not allow me to pass the realm of name and form. Again and again I tried to concentrate my mind upon the Advaita teachings, but every time the Mother's form stood in my way. In despair I said to "the naked one" (his Master Totapuri), "It is hopeless. I cannot raise my mind to the unconditioned state and come face to face with the Atman." He grew excited and sharply said, "What! You

can't do it? But you have to." He cast his eyes around for
something and finding a piece of glass he took it up and
pressing its point between my eyebrows said, "Concentrate your mind on this point." Then with stern determination I again sat to meditate, and as soon as the gracious form of the Divine Mother appeared before me, I
used my discrimination as a sword and with it severed it
into two. There remained no more obstruction to my
mind, which at once soared beyond the relative plane,
and I lost myself in Samadhi.*

It is clear therefore that while the bhakta can go very far
spiritually, can greatly enhance his consciousness, gain miracu-
lous powers, and anchored in a higher love rise above the love
of this world, it is nevertheless not possible for him to get
beyond the plane of "name and form," and therefore of relativity. He may get lost in the contemplation of the Godhead
with His amazing attributes, but he cannot experience the
same in its *Nirguna* and its *Anami,* its "Unconditioned" and
"Nameless" state. He can feel himself saturated with Cosmic
Consciousness, but it comes to him as something outside himself as a gift of grace, and he is not able to lose himself in It
and become one with the Ocean of Being. If he does seek to
attain that state, his accomplishment as a bhakta, instead of
helping him further, tends to hinder and obstruct him.

The two things that emerge from an examination of the
popular forms of yoga that were evolved after Patanjali are:
first that the soul can rise above physical consciousness, given
means whereby it can focus its energies, without recourse to
the arduous control of pranas, and second that full spiritual
realization or true samadhi is not merely a matter of transcending the physical (though that is necessary as a first step),
but is the end of a complex inner journey in which there are
many intermediate stages the attainment of which, under cer-

* *Sayings of Sri Ramakrishna* (Mylapore-Madras, 1954), page 313.

tain conditions, may be mistaken for the final goal and may thus debar further progress. The problem that arises before the true seeker in the face of such a situation is to discover a means other than that of pranas, jnana, or bhakti of an Isht-deva, as not only to enable the spirit-currents to be released from their present physical bondage, but also to enable the soul to be drawn upward unhindered from one spiritual plane to another until it transcends completely all the realms of relativity of *naam* and *rup,* of *kala* and *mahakala,* and reaches its goal: at-one-ment with the Nameless and Formless One.

The Sound Current

It is in the context of this problem that Surat Shabd Yoga, or the yoga of the celestial Sound Current, assumes its unique importance. Those who have mastered this yoga teach that the Absolute, though free of attributes in Its primal state, projects itself into form and assumes two primary attributes: Light and Sound. It is no mere accident, they point out, that in the revelatory literature of all major religions there are frequent references to the "Word" which occupies a central position in their pattern. In the Gospels we have:

> *In the beginning was the Word and the Word was*
> *with God and the Word was God.*

ST. JOHN

In ancient Indian scriptures we read repeatedly of *Aum,* the sacred Word pervading the three realms of bhur, bhuva and swah (i.e., the physical, astral and causal).

Again, Nanak says:

> *The earth and sky are of naught but Shabd (Word).*
> *From Shabd alone the light was born,*
> *From Shabd alone creation came,*
> *Shabd is the essential core in all.*

*Shabd is the directive agent of God, the cause of all
creation.*

PRABHATI

The Muslim Sufis declare:
*Creation came into being from Saut (Sound or
Word) and from Saut spread all light.*

SHAMAS TABREZ

*The Great Name is the very essence and life of all
   names and forms.*
Its manifest form sustains creation;
*It is the great ocean of which we are merely the
   waves,*
*He alone can comprehend this who has mastered
   our discipline.*

ABDUL RAZAQ KASHI

Moses heard the commandments of God amidst thunder
and flame, while in Zoroastrian and Taoist thought alike there
are references to the "Creative Verbum," the "Divine Light,"
and to the "Wordless Word," the silent Word.

Some learned scholars and theologians in subsequent times,
because of their own limited experience, have interpreted these
descriptions as metaphoric references to intuitive or intellectual
enlightenment. On closer examination such a position will be
found to be untenable. The terms "Word" or *Logos* as used
by the Greeks, Hebrews and Europeans, may be distorted to
mean "reason" or "order," and "light," may even be made to
mean no more than mental illumination, but their equivalents
in other religious literature—*nad, udgit, akash-bani, shabd,
naam, saut, bang-i-Ilahi, nida-i-asmani, sraosha, tao,* and
jyoti, prakash, tajalli, nur-i-yazdani, etc., refuse to bear such a
travesty of their original mystic meaning. What is more, some
seers have stated their real connotation in such a way that
there can be no scope for equivocation or room for doubt that

what is involved is not figurative expression of ordinary mental experience, but transcendent inner perception. Thus, in the Revelation of St. John we have:

> *His eyes were as a flame of fire . . . His voice as the sound of many waters . . . His countenance was as the sun shineth in his strength . . .*
> *And I heard a Voice from heaven, as the voice of many waters, and as the voice of a great thunder: and I heard the voice of harpers, harping with their harps.*

While in the Upanishads we are told:

> *First the murmuring sounds resembling those of the waves of the ocean, the fall of rain and then running rivulets, after which the bhervi will be heard, intermingled with the sounds of bell and conch.*

NAD BIND UPANISHAD

The Prophet Mohammad heard celestial music which gradually assumed the shape of Gabriel and formed itself into words; while Baha U'llah relates:

> *Myriads of mystic tongues find utterance in one speech, and myriads of His hidden mysteries are revealed in a single melody; yet alas, there is no ear to hear nor heart to understand!*
> *Blind thine eyes, that thou mayest behold My Beauty, and stop thine ears that thou mayest hearken unto the sweet melody of My Voice.*

These references to Light and Sound, say the Masters of the Surat Shabd Yoga, are not figurative but literal, referring not to the outer illuminations or sounds of this world, but to inner transcendent ones. They teach that the transcendent Sound and Light are the primal manifestations of God when He projects Himself into creation. In His Nameless state He is neither light nor darkness, neither sound nor silence, but when He assumes shape and form, Light and Sound emerge as His primary attributes.

This spirit force, Word, *Naam, Kalma* or God-in-action, is responsible for all that is, and the physical universes that we know are not the only ones that It has created. It has brought into being myriad regions and myriad creations over and above the physical. Indeed the whole is a grand unfathomable illimitable pattern in which the Positive pole (*Sach Khand* or *Sat Lok*) is a plane of pure, unalloyed spirit, while the Negative pole (*Pind*) is of gross physical matter with which we in this world are familiar. In between are countless regions which those who have journeyed from one end to the other often divide into three distinct planes in accordance with the balance of Positive-spiritual and Negative-material forces in each plane.

The Masters teach that the one constant principle that links all these planes from pure spirit to gross matter is the principle of the flaming sound or the sounding flame. The Word or *Shabd* as it descends downward assumes a varying density of spirituo-material forces. Mystics speak of the purple light and the light of the noonday or setting sun, and refer to the sounds of flutes, harps, violins, conches, thunder, bells, running water, etc., but though manifesting differently at different levels the *Shabd* yet remains constant in Itself.

As a river springing from the snowy peak of a towering mountain flows toward the sea, it undergoes many changes of setting, shape, motion and appearance, and yet its waters remain the same.

If one could discover this audible life-stream within oneself, if one could discover its lower reaches, one could use it as a pathway leading inevitably to its source. The currents might at certain points enter gorges and rapids, but nevertheless they

are the surest way on the upward journey. Be a range howsoever unscalable, the waters will have cut a pass and carved
a passage, and he who will avail himself of their guidance
would never fail to find a way. And since this *Naam* or Word-
current springs from the *Anaam* or the Wordless, he who
holds firmly to It will inevitably reach the starting point, transcending plane after plane of varying relativity until he arrives
at the very source of name and form; thence to merge into
That which has no name or form.

The cornerstones

The Sound Current undoubtedly offers the surest way to
man for reaching from form to the Formless, but the question
arises, how can man get access to It and thus accomplish his
inner journey? Those proficient in this path always maintain
that there are three conditions that must be fulfilled before
success in this truest of all yogas can be attained:

Satguru: The first condition is that of finding a Satguru or
true teacher who is an adept in this mystic science. The subject
is one of practical self-realization, not of philosophic disserta-
tion or intuitive feeling. If it were one of mere theory, then
books and scriptures would be enough for our purpose, and
if it were one of mere feeling then each could trust the
promptings of his own mind. But the question before us is
that of unlocking a "sixth" sense, one of direct transcendental
perception, of inner hearing and seeing. One born deaf and
blind may, with the help of Braille, learn the most detailed
expositions of man's rich and varied audio-visual experiences,
but his study can never give him direct experience. The most
that he can get from books is the realization of an extensive
plane of experience wholly beyond him, and this can generate
in him the urge to discover means whereby he can overcome
his physical limitations. It is the expert surgeon or doctor who

alone can effect a cure (provided his ailment is curable). And should he fall into the hands of a charlatan, his condition will only become worse and more complicated.

In like manner, the aspirant who seeks inner spiritual mastery must seek the aid of one who has already mastered the way. All his readings of scriptures, all his thinking, can at best lead to a single conclusion, provided he is sensitive to the point involved: the need for a living Master. Without such a Master he cannot even understand the true import of the revelatory scriptures. They speak of experiences beyond his level of experience, and even in his own language they can only speak in metaphors and parables, for how can the discourses of the blind be made to express directly that of the seeing? To attempt to interpret the rich spiritual heritage in our religious literature wholly in terms of our own limited experience might lead to a distortion of the true meaning. We might gather a great deal of psychological wisdom, but the inner significance would be lost on us, and all our intellectual theorizing would only land us in unending theological contradictions with which the various institutionalized religions are encumbered today.

Only one who has himself experienced what the great scriptures describe, can guide us to their real significance. But the task of a spiritual teacher does not end there. The elucidation of the true meaning of religion is no more than a first step. After the aspirant has understood the nature of his goal, he must pursue it practically and rationally. To know is one thing, and to do is quite another. It is only after he has explained to the aspirant the end to be attained that the Master's real task begins. It is not enough that the doctor diagnoses the cause of the blind man's ailment, he must perform the operation as well. So too the spiritual guide at the time of initiation gives the disciple a first-hand experience of the inner Light and Sound. He puts him into touch with the Divine Stream, be it at its lowest level, and instructs him in the sadhnas to be followed for consolidating and developing this inner experience to its full extent.

He who can find such a teacher is blessed indeed. But to discover such a one and be initiated by him is not enough. The germinal spiritual experience that he gives must be nurtured and developed to the point of full spiritual efflorescence. To be able to do this, one must accept whatever one learns and attempt to put it into practice. To know such a man is to love him, and to love him is to follow his commandments. Until one can thus love and obey, and so transform one's life, the gift of the Guru remains as a seed locked away in a steel vault where it cannot sprout and grow to fruition.

Sadachar: It is the necessity for self-discipline that makes sadachar the second cornerstone of the pattern. The word *sadachar* is not easy to translate. One can find many literal equivalents, but none of them really expresses its extensive and many-sided significance. In brief, it stands for the good and pure life. It does not imply any rigid code or set moral formulae, but suggests purity and simplicity, which radiate from within and spread outwards, permeating every action, every word, every thought. It is as much concerned with one's personal habits, good and hygienic, as with one's individual and social ethics. And on its ethical side, it is concerned not merely with one's relation to one's fellow men but to all living things, i.e., harmony which is the result of recognition that all things are from the same Essence, and so a worm is as much a part of Brahman as the mightiest of gods, Indra.

The first lesson taught by a true Guru is that of "the identity of substance," and he who has grasped this truth will discipline his life accordingly. He will not be a prey to inordinate desires, and his one aim will be to reach the still point which holds in itself all actions, the point where to have nothing is to possess everything. He will know that the one path to fulfillment is through renunciation, and the one way to reach the Almighty is through freeing himself from all other attachments:

> *In order to arrive at having pleasure in everything,*
> *Desire to have pleasure in nothing.*
> *In order to arrive at possessing everything,*
> *Desire to possess nothing.*
> *In order to arrive at being everything,*
> *Desire to be nothing.*
>
> ST. JOHN OF THE CROSS

> *Cleanse the chamber of thy heart*
> *That thy Beloved may enter.*
>
> TULSI SAHIB

> *Where there is nothing, there is God.*
>
> W. B. YEATS

Freed from the demon of desire (*kama*), he will be freed from the demon of wrath (*krodh*), which follows upon frustration of desire. Liberated from these, he would be freed also from greed (*lobh*), attachment (*moh*) and pride (*ahankar*), which are but the extensions of desire.

His would be a life of detachment or of *nishkama*. But detachment would not be for him a life of indifference or of ascetic renunciation. To know all life is to discover a new bond between oneself and the rest of creation. He who knows this cannot be merely "indifferent." He must perforce be filled to overflowing with sympathy for all that he confronts, and sympathy toward the whole must imply a certain holy indifference to the part. He will no longer be tied to his own narrow individual interests, but will share his love and resources with all. He will develop, slowly but surely, something of the compassion of the Buddha and the love of Christ. Nor will he feel himself called upon to leave the world for the solitude of the forest, the mountain or the desert cave. The detachment must be an inner one, and one who cannot achieve it at home will not achieve it in the forest. He will recognize the great use of occasional retreats from worldly affairs and cares to the silence of solitary meditation and concentration, but he will not seek to escape from life and its responsibilities. He will be a loving husband and a good father, but while being these he will never forget the ultimate purpose of life, always knowing how to give unto Caesar that which is Caesar's, and preserving for God that which is God's. The way for transcending desire, he will know, is not through repressing it but meeting it squarely and overcoming it. To him, *sanyasa* is not a matter of outer evasion or escapism but of inner freedom, an idea that is well expressed by Nanak thus:

> *Let contentment be your ear-rings,*
> *And endeavor for the Divine and respect for the*
>   *higher Self your wallet,*
> *And constant meditation on Him your ashes,*
> *Let preparedness for death be your cloak,*
> *And let your body be like unto a chaste virgin.*
> *Let your Master's teachings be your supporting*
>   *staff.*
>
> JAP JI

The two cardinal virtues that such a man will cultivate will be charity and chastity. He will be large of heart and bounteous, caring more for the sufferings of others than for his own, and easily forgiving those that injure him. He will be simple and restrained in his habits. His wants will be few and easily satisfied, for one who has too many desires and too many attachments cannot be pure of heart. For him chastity will extend even to giving up meat and drink. When all life is one, to live upon the flesh of other living beings would be to defile oneself. And when one's goal is to attain even higher realms of consciousness, to resort to narcotics and intoxicants is only to court regression. It is not an idiosyncracy of Indian seers that they should have made abstinence from meat and drink a necessary part of the spiritual discipline. We have similar injunctions in the Koran and the Holy Bible. Thus in Proverbs 23:20, we find:

> Be not among winebibbers; among riotous eaters of flesh.

And in Romans 14:21:

> It is good neither to eat flesh, nor to drink wine, nor anything whereby thy brother stumbleth, or is offended, or is made weak.

And in I Corinthians 6:13:

> Meats for the belly, and belly for meats; but God shall destroy both it and them. Now the body is not for fornication but for the Lord; and the Lord for the body.

In the *Essene Gospel of John* (direct translation from the Aramaic of the pure original words of Jesus), we have:

But they answered Him: "Whither should we go, Master, . . . for with you are the words of eternal life. Tell us, what are the sins we must shun, that we may nevermore see disease?"

Jesus answered: "Be it so according to your faith," and He sat down among them, saying:

"It was said to them of olden time, 'Honor thy Heavenly Father and thy Earthly Mother, and their commandments, that thy days may be long upon the earth.' And next was given this commandment: 'Thou shalt not kill,' for life is given to all by God, and that which God has given, let not man take away. For I tell you truly, from one Mother proceeds all that lives upon the earth. Therefore he who kills, kills his brother. And from him will the Earthly Mother turn away, and will pluck from him her quickening breasts. And he will be shunned by her angels, and Satan will have his dwelling in his body. And the flesh of slain beasts in his body will become his own tomb. For I tell you truly, he who kills, kills himself, and whosoever eats the flesh of slain beasts, eats of the body of death. And their death will become his death. For the wages of sin is death. Kill not, neither eat the flesh of your innocent prey, lest you become the slaves of Satan. For that is the path of sufferings, and it leads unto death. But do the Will of God, that his angels may serve you on the way of life. Obey, therefore, the words of God: 'Behold, I have given you every herb, bearing seed, which is upon the face of all the earth, and every tree, in which is the fruit of a tree yielding seed; to you it shall be for meat. And to every beast of the earth, and to every fowl of the air, and to everything that creepeth upon the earth wherein there is breath of life, I give every green herb for meat.' Also the milk of everything that moveth and that liveth upon each shall be meat for you; even as the green herb have I given unto them, so I give their milk unto you. But flesh, and the blood which quickens it, shall ye not eat."

And Jesus continued: "God commanded your fore-fathers, 'Thou shalt not kill.' But their heart was hardened and they killed. Then Moses desired that at least they should not kill men, and he suffered them to kill beasts. And then the heart of your forefathers was hardened yet more, and they killed men and beasts likewise. But I say to you: Kill neither men, nor beasts, nor yet the food which goes into your mouth. For if you eat living food the same will quicken you, but if you kill your food, the dead food will kill you also. For life comes only from life, and from death comes always death. For everything which kills your foods, kills your bodies also. And everything which kills your bodies, kills your souls also. And your bodies become what your foods are, even as your spirits, likewise, become what your thoughts are."

With the chastity in food and drink will go another kind of chastity, the one that pertains to sex. One will not suppress all sexual desire, for repression can only breed neurosis and prepare the way for a downfall, but he will be ever seeking to sublimate it. He will understand that nature's purpose in this instinct is to preserve the race and will channel it so as to fulfill that purpose, never making it an end in itself, a source of physical pleasure, for when it becomes that, it turns into a drug that anaesthetizes the spirit and begins to defeat nature's purpose of procreation by encouraging the invention and use of contraceptives.

In short, the sincere and conscientious aspirant will reorient his entire mode of life, in eating and drinking, thinking, acting, feeling, etc. He will gradually weed out of his mind all irrelevant and unhealthy desires, until he gradually attains the state of purity and simplicity that marks the child.

> *Verily I say unto you, except ye be converted and become as little children, ye shall not enter into the Kingdom of God.*
>
> ST. MATTHEW

All religious teachers the world over, laid great stress on higher moral values, and these in fact, constitute the groundwork for their teachings. A true Master always insists on the maintaining of a record of daily lapses in thought, word and deed, from non-injury, truth, chastity, universal love and selfless service of all, the five cardinal virtues that pave the way for spirituality. It is only the knowledge of our faults that can make us weed them out and strive in the right direction.

Through all this process of reintegration, his inspiration will be the example of his Master and the inner experience he gives. His Master's life will be a living testament beckoning him toward the ideal of sadachar, and the experience he has of the Word within will stand as a proof of the truth of what his Master teaches. Sadachar is no dry discipline that can be attained by following certain set formulae. It is a way of life, and in such matters only heart to heart can speak. It is this that makes Satsang, or association with a true Master, so important. It not only serves as a constant reminder of the goal before the seeker, but through the magic touch of personal contact, gradually transforms his entire mode of thinking and feeling. As his heart and mind under this benign influence grow gradually purer, his life more fully centers in the divine. In short, as he increasingly realizes in practice the ideal of sadachar, his thoughts, now scattered and dissipated, will gain equipoise and integration till they arrive at so fine a focus that the veils of inner darkness are burnt to cinders and the inner glory stands revealed.

Sadhna: And now we come to the third cornerstone of the spiritual edifice, that of spiritual sadhna or discipline. The one recurrent theme of a *puran guru* or perfect teacher, is that the good life, though highly desirable and indispensable, is not an end in itself. The goal of life is something inner and different. It is an ascension from the plane of relativity and physical existence into one of Absolute Being. He who recognizes this will mould his life accordingly, first, because such a recognition implies a state of mind that, being free from ego and attachment, expesses itself in virtuous and creative action, and second, because without cultivating such a state of mind and of life one cannot attain the poise and concentration required for inner ascension.

So the basic stress of the enlightened teacher is laid always upon the transcendental goal. He teaches that the pranic and vigyanic energies are not of the essence of Atman, but take their birth in planes lower than those of pure spirit. He who

would use them as a ladder may transcend bodily consciousness, may reach the planes whence they originate, but he cannot reach beyond. The spirit being similar in all, the means
to spiritual enlightenment should likewise be accessible to all.
But, as has been seen already, such forms of yoga as are based
on the pranas or on jnana make special demands which all
cannot fulfill. The pranic systems are beyond the reach of the
old or those of tender years, and also of those who suffer from
any respiratory or digestive disorders. The path of jnana pre-
sumes mental and intellectual capacities that Nature bestows
only on few. If these approaches were indeed the natural ones
open to us, then the logical conclusion would be that Nature
is very partial in her blessings, discriminating between man
and man. Why, if the sun shines for all, and the wind blows
for all, should the inner treasures be available only to the
chosen few? They are also for the learned and the unlearned.

Yogas that are so discriminating in selecting their practitioners, and so exacting in their practice, cannot be wholly
natural. The method taught by the Masters of the Surat
Shabd Yoga is different. As mentioned earlier, the nature of
creation and the way back to life's initial source is explained
to the seeker. At the time of initiation, he is given a first-hand
inner experience which he is taught to develop. The seat of
the soul is between and behind the eyebrows. This at least is
accepted by all yogas. It is to this point that mystics refer
when they speak of *shiv netra, divya chakshu, tisra til, Brahm-
rendra, triambka, trilochana, nukta-i-sweda, koh-i-toor,* third
eye, single eye, figuratively called the still point, the mount of
transfiguration, etc. It is at this point that the sadhak having
closed his eyes must focus his attention, but the effort at concentration must be an effortless one and there must be no
question of any physical or mental strain. To assist this effort
the teacher gives the disciple a *mantra,* or charged verbal
formula, which is symbolic of the journey ahead. This for-

mula, when repeated slowly and lovingly with the tongue of thought, helps the disciple to collect his scattered thoughts gradually at a single point. What gives this mantra its potency is not any magic inherent in the words per se, but the fact that it is given by one who, by his own spiritual practice and mastery, has charged it with inner power. When the aspirant, by his inner concentration and by the mental repetition of the charged words, has brought his inward gaze to a sharp and steady focus, he will find that the darkness within that he at first confronted, gets gradually illuminated by shifting points of light. As his powers of concentration increase, the lights cease flickering and develop into a single radiating point.

This process of concentration, or the collection of *surat,* automatically draws the spirit-currents, normally dissipated all over the body, toward the spiritual center. This withdrawal is greatly assisted by *simran* or repetition of the charged mantra; and the perception of the inner light, leading to *dhyan* or one-pointed concentration, quickens the process still further. In turn, dhyan when fully developed, leads to *bhajan* or inner hearing. The inner light begins to become resonant.

Within thee is Light and within the Light the Sound,
and the same shall keep thee attached to the True
One.

GURBANI

The practitioner, when he shuts his physical ears, gets rapidly absorbed into the music. It is a common experience that though light can catch the eye, it cannot hold it for very long and has no very magnetic quality about it. But with music it is different. He who hears it in silence and stillness, is drawn irresistibly, as it were, into another world, a different realm of experience. And so the process of withdrawal that begins with simran, is stimulated by dhyan, and is rapidly extended by bhajan. The spiritual currents, already moving slowly, are

carried upward, collecting finally at the third eye—the seat
of the soul. The spiritual transcending of physical consciousness, or death in life, is thus achieved with the minimum of
effort and travail.

When students of the other forms of yoga reach the state
of full physical transcendence after a long and exacting mastery of the lower chakras, they generally assume that they
have reached their journey's end. The inner plane at which
they find themselves—the realm of Sahasrar or Sahasdal
Kamal, often symbolised by the sun-wheel, the lotus or the
multifoliate rose—is indeed incomparably more beautiful
than anything on earth, and in comparison appears timeless.
But when the student of the Surat Shabd Yoga succeeds in
rising above physical consciousness, he finds the Radiant Form
of his Master waiting unsought to receive him. Indeed, it is at
this point that the real *Guru-shishya* or teacher-student relationship is established. Up to this stage, the Guru had been
little more than a human teacher, but now he is seen as the
divine guide or *Gurudev,* who shows the inner way:

> *The feet of my Master have been manifested in my*
> *   forehead,*
> *And all my wanderings and tribulations have ended.*
>
> GURU ARJAN

> *With the appearance of the Radiant Form of the*
> *Master within,*
> *No secret remains hidden in the womb of time.*

Christ also speaks in the same strain:

> *There is nothing covered, that shall not be revealed,*
> *and hid, that shall not be known.*
>
> ST. MATTHEW

Under the guidance of this Celestial Guide the soul learns
to overcome the first shock of joy, and realizes that its goal lies

still far ahead. Accompanied by the Radiant Form and drawn by the Audible Life Current, it traverses from region to region, from plane to plane, dropping off kosha after kosha, until at last it stands wholly divested of all that is not of its nature. Thus disentangled and purified it can at last enter the realm where it sees that it is of the same essence as the Supreme Being, that the Master in His Radiant Form and the soul are not separate but One, and that there is naught but the Great Ocean of Consciousness, of Love, of Bliss ineffable. Who shall describe the splendor of this realm?

> *Only heart to heart can speak of the bliss of mystic knowers:*
> *No messenger can tell it and no missive bear it.*
>
> HAFIZ

> *When the pen set to picturing this station,*
> *It broke in pieces and the page was torn.*
>
> PERSIAN MYSTIC

Having reached the journey's end, the seeker too merges with the Word and enters the company of the Free Ones. He may continue to live like other men in this world of human beings, but his spirit knows no limitations and is as infinite as God Himself. The wheel of transmigration can no longer affect him, and his consciousness knows no restrictions. Like his Master before him, he has become a Conscious Co-worker of the Divine Plan. He does nothing for himself but works in God's name. If there be indeed any *Neh-Karmi* (one free from the bonds of action), it is he, for there is no more potent means to freedom than the Power of the Word.

> *He alone is action-free who communes with the Word.*
>
> GURBANI

Freedom for him is not something that comes after death (*videh mukti*); it is something achieved in life itself. He is a *jivan-mukta* (free-in-life); like a flower shedding fragrance, he spreads the message of freedom wherever he goes.

> *Those who have communed with the Word, their*
> *toils shall end.*
> *And their faces shall flame with glory.*
> *Not only shall they have salvation,*
> *O Nanak, but many more shall find freedom with*
> *them.*

JAP JI

In actual practice of the spiritual discipline, stress is laid on *Simran, Dhyan* and *Bhajan,* each of which plays a specific role in unfoldment of the Self. The Master gives Simran or mental repetition of the charged words, which help in gathering together the wandering wits of the practitioner to the still point of the soul between and behind the two eyebrows, to which place the sensory currents now pervading from top to toe are withdrawn, and one becomes lost to the consciousness of the flesh. The successful completion of this process of itself leads to dhyan or concentration. Dhyan is derived from the Sanskrit root *dhi,* meaning "to bind" and "to hold on." With the inner eye opened, the aspirant now sees shimmering streaks of heaven's light within him and this keeps his attention anchored. Gradually, the light grows steady in his sadhna, for it works as a sheet-anchor for the soul. Dhyan or concentration when perfected, leads one to *Bhajan* or attuning to the music which emerges from within the center of the holy light. This enchanting holy melody has a magnetic pull which is irresistible, and the soul cannot but follow it to the spiritual source from whence the music emerges. The soul is helped by this triple process to slide out of the shackles of the body and becomes anchored in the heavenly radiance of its Self (atman), and is led on to the heavenly home of the Father.

The entire process is nurtured by *Sat Naam, Satguru* and *Satsang,* which in fact are synonymous for the Master Power at work. Sat Naam is the Power of the Absolute stirred into compassion and when It puts on the flesh, It assumes the form of the Guru (Word made flesh), and works through him by means of Satsang, both outer and inner, which helps the jivas ripe for regeneration. This Power works on all the planes simultaneously, according to the needs of each individual; by word of mouth as a Guru in human form, sharing in all joys and sorrows of the human beings; by inner guidance as Gurudeva in his astral, luminous or radiant form, and finally as Satguru—a veritable Master of Truth.

There are two ways within: *jyoti marg* and *sruti marg* (the way of light and the way of sound), respectively. The holy Light keeps the soul anchored and absorbed and to a certain extent leads the soul as well, but the holy Word pulls it upward and carries it across from plane to plane in spite of various hurdles on the Way, like blinding or bewildering lights, densely pitch darkness, etc., until the soul reaches its destination.

A perfect science

Even the foregoing bird's-eye survey of the nature and scope of the Surat Shabd Yoga conveys some of its unique features. He who studies it in relation to the other forms of yoga cannot but note the completeness of its solution of all the problems that confront the seeker when pursuing other systems. On the plane of outer action, it does not base itself on a dry and rigid discipline that is often laden with the consequences of psychological repression. It holds that some discipline is necessary, but adds that it must ultimately be inspired by inner spiritual experience and be a matter of spontaneous living, and not of rigorous asceticism and a too deliberate self abnegation. The seeker must strive toward a state of equipoise and must therefore cultivate the virtue of moderation in thought and deed. The integration he thereby achieves enables him to gain greater concentration, and so higher inner experience, and this inner experience must in turn have repercussions on outer thoughts and action. The relationship of sadachar to inner sadhna is a reciprocal one; each enlivens and gives meaning to the other, and one without the other is like a bird with a single wing. How can the spirit be brought to perfect one-pointedness without the purity of mind and body, and how can the soul transcend all human attachments and imperfections without centering itself in the love of the Divine?

> *When the qualities of the Ancient of Days stood revealed,*
> *Then the qualities of earthly things did Moses burn away.*
>
> RUMI

The Surat Shabd Yoga not only provides a means for achieving in practice the difficult ideal of sadachar, it also offers a mode of life that, while raising one above this physical world, does not enslave one to the realm of Name and Form. The Masters of this path know only too well that abstract speculations about the non-attributive aspect of the Absolute cannot lead one to It. How can man, conditioned by name and form, be drawn directly to that which is beyond name or form? Love seeks something which it can comprehend and to which it can attach itself, and God, if He is to meet man, must assume some shape or form. It is this recognition that inspires the devotion of the bhakta to Shiva, Vishnu, Krishna, or Kali, the Divine Mother. But these divine beings represent fixed manifestations of God, and once the devotee has reached their plane, their very fixity, as we have seen already, prevents further progress. The Masters of the Surat Shabd Yoga wholly transcend this limitation by linking the seeker not to a fixed, but to an all-pervading manifestation of God; the Radiant Sound Current. It is this *anhat* and *anhad* Naam, this un-struck and unfathomable Word, that supports the various planes of creation ranging from pure spirit to gross matter. Its strains pervade every realm, every region, and it runs through them like a river that flows through the valleys which it has brought into being. And like the river, it exists in a fluid state, changing at every plane, yet ever remaining the same. The seeker who has been inspired by the love of the river of the Word is blessed indeed for he knows none of the limitations experienced by those who adore God in other forms. As he is drawn upward by Its beatific power, he finds It changing, modifying, becoming even stronger and purer, beckoning him on to higher and still higher effort, never allowing him to halt or to loiter, but leading him on from plane to plane, from valley to valley, until he arrives at the very source from where the Unmanifested comes into manifestation, the Formless as-sumes form, and the Nameless, name. It was this completeness of the inner journey made possible by the Yoga of the Sound Current that led Kabir to declare:

> *All holy ones are worthy of reverence,*
> *But I adore only one who has mastered the Word.*

The Surat Shabd Yoga is not only the most perfect of the various yogas, but it is also comparatively easy to practice, and one accessible to all. Not only do those following this path reach the ultimate end, but they do so with greater economy of effort than is possible by the other methods. The transcend-ence of physical consciousness that the yogin pursuing the path of the pranas achieves only after a long and arduous dis-cipline, is attained by practitioners of the Surat Shabd Yoga sometimes at the first sitting at the time of initiation. That this should be so is not a mere chance or accident. The fact is that the Surat Shabd Yoga adopts a more scientific and natural approach to man's spiritual problems. Why, it asserts, if the spiritual current reaches the bodily chakras not from below but from above, should it be necessary to master each of these chakras in turn? A man standing at the heart of a valley, if he wishes to reach the river's source, does not have to travel down to its mouth and then retraverse the distance. It further holds that if prana and mind (even at their most refined) are not of the true essence of the spirit, then how can they be the best means of disengaging it from its encrustations? If it could be put in touch with that which is of its own essential nature, like would draw like, and with the minimum of effort the desired end would be achieved. It is from the point of the *tisra-til,* the third eye, that the spiritual current spreads itself into the body. All that is needed is to check its downward flow at this point by controlling one's senses and it would, of its own accord, collect itself and flow backwards toward its source.

> *Shutter your lip, your ear, your eye*
> *And if you do not Truth descry,*
> *Then let your scorn upon me fly.*
>
> HAFIZ

The seeker has no need to begin from the very bottom, all he has to do is to turn in the direction of the spiritual stream and the rest will follow.

> *What is there in reaching the Lord?*
> *One needs only to transplant the heart.*
>
> INAYAT SHAH

It is this simplicity of approach coupled with economy of effort that has induced many to call the Surat Shabd Yoga the *Sehaj Marg* or the Easy Way. It begins at the point where other yogas normally tend to end. Sahasrar, the region of the thousand-petaled lights, which marks the end of the normal yogin's journey after traversing the various bodily chakras, is well-nigh the first step to be taken by the follower of the Surat Shabd Yoga. Further, by refusing to disturb the pranic or kundalinic energies, this yoga greatly reduces the strain of physical transcendence. By contacting the Sound-principle, the sensory currents are automatically drawn upward without the practitioner consciously striving to achieve this end, and the motor currents are left untouched. Not only does this simplify the process of entry into the state of samadhi, but that of returning from it as well. The adept in this path needs no outer assistance for coming back into physical consciousness, as is the case with some other yogic forms; spiritual ascension and descent are entirely voluntary and can be achieved by him with the rapidity of thought.

The method of transcendental hearing is only an extension of our normal daily practice. When we are faced with some knotty problem, our entire conscious energies tend to focus at one point—the seat of the soul—without affecting pranic-motor energies functioning automatically in our body. The Surat Shabd Yoga practitioner achieves this concentration at will under controlled conditions through simran and dhyan, and as soon as he contacts the reverberating Word, the sensory spiritual current that is still in the body is drawn irresistibly upward and complete physical transcendence is achieved.

It is this quality of *sehaj,* of naturalness and ease, that makes the Surat Shabd Yoga accessible to all. The music of the Divine Word is vibrating in all alike, and he who follows Its path, needs no special requirements, whether physical or intellectual. It is as much open to the old as to the young, to the sinners as to the saints, to the simple as to the learned, to women and children as to men. Indeed, women and children and the unsophisticated, owing to their simpler modes of thought and their spontaneous faith, often make quicker initial headway with this method than their more sophisticated brethren. However, full attainment in this field demands unwavering perseverance and effort, which may not always be forthcoming. As no rigorous and extensive disciplines of food, physical exercises, etc., are required, it does not necessitate *sanyasa* or complete renunciation of the world, and is as much open to the *grehastis,* the married, as to the *brahmcharis,* those who are under a vow of celibacy. Had the pranic and vigyanic systems been the most natural available then we should have had to conclude Nature to be partial, for the physical and mental capabilities they require are distributed unequally among men. If the sun and the air are available to all, why should the spiritual gifts be reserved only for the chosen few? Besides, prana and vigyan can at best lead one to the plane of their origin and as they are not purely spiritual, how can they lead to the realm of pure spirit?

However, to say that the Surat Shabd Yoga is the most perfect of the yogic sciences and the most natural, is not to say that it demands no effort and that anyone can just take to it and succeed. Had that been the case, humanity would not have been floundering as it is today. The fact is that competent teachers of this crown of all sciences are rare and that even when a teacher is found, few are prepared to undergo the kind of discipline required. The spirit may be willing, but the flesh is weak. Most men are so deeply engrossed with the love of the world that even after having had a glimpse of inner treasures they are reluctant to give up their worldly ways and concentrate on the possession of that which makes one the master of all. Since the stress in this yoga is always on the inner, never on the outer, no path could in a way be more exacting for the general run of men. Many can spend whole lives in outer ritual and ceremonial but few can attain perfect inner concentration, undisturbed by mundane thoughts, even for a few moments. Hence it was that Kabir compared it to walking on a naked sword, while the Sufis spoke of it as the *rah-i-mustqim,* finer than a hair and sharper than the razor's edge. Christ described it as the "strait and narrow way" that only a few ever tread. But for one whom the world lures not and who is filled with a passionate love of God, nothing could be easier and quicker. He needs no other force than that of his own urge and, purified of earthly attachments by his sincere and strong longing, his soul shall wing homeward, borne on the stream of Shabd toward its point of origin, the haven of bliss and peace. Should the soul confront any obstacles on its homing flight, its Radiant Friend is always beside it to lead it past and protect it from all pitfalls.

The road through the higher planes lies charted before the soul as completely as that for Hatha yogins of the lower bodily chakras, and with such a Power to bear it, and such a Friend to guide, nothing can deter or entrap, nothing can disturb the steadiness of its course. "Take hold of the garment, O brave soul, of One who knows well all places, physical, mental, supra-mental and spiritual, for he will remain thy friend in life as well as in death, in this world and the worlds beyond," exhorted Jalalud-din Rumi.

And sang Nanak:

> *He that has found a True Master and pursues the perfect way of the Holy Word shall, laughing and living in this world, find full freedom and emancipation.*

Again,

> *Like the lotus shall he rise immaculate above the mire of the world and like the swan shall he shoot forth from its murky waters untouched and untrammelled.*

The Master

Apart from its scientific approach, its comparatively easy accessibility, its quality of naturalness and its freedom from the drawbacks of other yogic forms, another distinctive feature of the Yoga of the Sound Current is the unique and pervasive emphasis it lays on the need at every step for a Satguru, *Pir-e-rah* or *Murshid-i-Kamil* (a competent, living Master). Though something on this theme has already been mentioned under "The cornerstones," much remains to be elaborated.

The *Guru-shish* or *Guru-sikh* relationship is important in all forms of practical yoga, but it is pivotal here in a unique sense. For the Guru in the Surat Shabd Yoga is not only a being who explains to us the real nature of existence, instructs us in the true values of life and tells us of the sadhnas to be practiced for inner attainment, he is all this and more. He is the inner guide as well, leading the soul from plane to plane to its ultimate destination, a guide without whose aid the soul would mistake the intermediate stages for the final goal and would encounter barriers which it would be unable to surmount.

The role of the Master being what it is, it is little wonder that all mystics who have pursued this way should have sung of him with superlative reverence and adoration. From Kabir, we read:

> *I wish and long for the dust of his feet — the dust*
> *that has created the universe;*
> *His lotus feet are the true wealth and a haven of*
> *peace.*
> *They grant ineffable wisdom and lead one on the*
> *path Godward.*

And the Sikh scriptures sing:

> *Sweet are the lotus feet of the Master;*
> *With God's writ one sees them;*

> *And myriad are the blessings that follow upon such*
> *a vision.*
>
> GURU ARJAN

From the Sufis, we have:

> *If I were to sing praises of his countless blessings till*
> *eternity,*
> *I could hardly say anything of them.*
>
> JALALUD-DIN RUMI

Some mystics even go to the extent of raising his position above that of God:

> *The Master is greater than God.*
>
> KABIR

> *The Guru and God both stand manifested, whom*
> *may I adore and render obeisance?*
> *Wonderful indeed is the Guru who has revealed the*
> *God-power within.*
>
> SEHJO BAI

All this may lead the sceptic to suspect human idolatry. He may ask: "Why this deification of a human being? Why such praise heaped upon one who is mortal?" Mystics at times have responded to this question with holy indifference:

> *People decry that Khusro has turned idolator;*
> *Indeed I have, but what has the world to do with*
> *me?*
>
> AMIR KHUSRO

But sometimes, they have themselves answered it fully:

> *Without the munificence of the Master one gets*
> *naught,*
> *Even if one engages in a million meritorious deeds.*
>
> GURBANI

Devotion to God keeps one entangled in this (physi-
cal) life — just consider gravely,
But devotion to the Master carries one back unto
God.

KABIR

Enter within and verify for yourself,
Who is greater of the two: God or the Guru.

GURBANI

God drove me into the wilderness of the world, but
the Master has snapped for me the ceaseless chain
of transmigration.

SEHJO BAI

All great spiritual teachers have maintained that without
the help of a living Master, the spiritual journey is difficult
and impossible to traverse to the very end. Jalalud-din Rumi,
the Persian mystic, suggests this forcefully when he says:

Veiled from this was Moses
Though all strength and light,
Then thou who hast no wings at all,
Attempt not flight.

And makes his meaning still clearer elsewhere:

Find a Master spirit, for without his active help and
guidance, this journey is beset with dangers, perils
and fears.

In the Gospels it is the same strain that vibrates through
the sayings of Jesus:

No man cometh unto the Father but by me.

ST. JOHN

No man knoweth who the Father is, but the Son;
and he to whom the Son will reveal Him.

ST. LUKE AND ST. MATTHEW

No man can come to me, except the Father which
hath sent me draw him; and I will raise him up at
the last day.

ST. JOHN

While conferring apostleship on the twelve disciples, Jesus said unto them:

He that receiveth you receiveth me, and he that re-
ceiveth me receiveth Him that sent me.

Wherefore he was able to save them to the uttermost that came unto God by him, seeing he ever liveth to make intercession for them.

The Master is indeed the "Intercessor" or *Rasul,* who moves between us and God, linking us to the holy Word, and without him there could be but little hope of salvation. No friendship could be greater than his friendship, no love truer than his love, no gift greater than his grace. Chance winds may blow others apart and death may come to part the most faithful lovers; he alone is unfailing in life as well as in death:

I have commanded you; and, lo! I am with you
always, even unto the end of the world.

ST. MATTHEW

He alone is a friend who accompanies me on my
*   last journey,*
And shields me before the judgment seat of God.

GURBANI

Other gifts may decay and perish, but his gift, the gift of God's Word, is imperishable, indestructible, ever shining, ever fresh, ever new, a boon in life, a greater boon in death.

From where does the Master derive this unique and super-human power that makes him almost equal to God and, in the eyes of his disciples, places him even above God? Can mortal flesh compete with the Immortal and the finite outdistance the Infinite? This may well seem a paradox to the world, but those who have crossed with opened eyes to the inner Kingdom, see in this no contradiction, only the mystery of God's greatness. The true Master is one who under instruction and guidance from his own teacher has learned to analyze the soul from the body, has traversed the inner path to its very end, and has beheld the source of all light and life and merged with the Nameless One. After merging with the Nameless One, he becomes one with Him and one with all that is. On the human plane he may appear as limited as any one of us, but on the spiritual, he is Limitless and Infinite even as God Himself:

O my servant obey Me, and I shall make thee like unto Myself. I say, "Be," and it is, and thou shalt say "Be," and it shall be.

BAHA'U'LLAH — THE FOUR VALLEYS

The Word was made flesh, and dwelt amongst us.

ST. JOHN

The Word is the Master and the Prophet, full of wisdom deep and profound.

GURU NANAK

When I churned the sea of body, a strange truth came to light,
God was identified in the Master and no distinction could Nanak find.

GURU RAM DAS

Guru is Brahma, Guru is Vishnu, Guru is Shiva and Guru is the veritable Par-Brahm, and we offer our salutation to Him.

The Guru-shish relationship has very often been described as below:

> *Who is the true Guru for a disciple?*
> *Shabd indeed is the Guru and Surat the disciple of*
> *the Dhun (Sound).*

GURU NANAK

> *The Shabd-Guru is too deep and unfathomable,*
> *Without (the Controlling Power of) the Shabd the*
> *world would be but a wilderness.*

GURU NANAK

> *The Word of the Master is Master indeed, full of*
> *life-giving water,*
> *He who follows His Word doth verily cross the*
> *strands of time.*

GURU RAM DAS

> *The disciple-Surat can traverse the Path only with*
> *the Shabd-Guru,*
> *Exploring the heavenly mysteries, it doth find rest*
> *in the inverted well (of the head).*

TULSI SAHIB

> *Know it for certain that Shabd-Guru is the veritable*
> *Guru,*
> *Surat can truly become the disciple of the Dhun by*
> *being a Gur-mukh (receptacle for the Word).*

BHAI GURDAS

> *Guru resides in the gagan (spiritual realm above)*
> *and the disciple in the ghat (between the two*
> *eyebrows).*
> *When the two, the Surat and the Shabd, do meet,*
> *they get united eternally.*

KABIR

SURAT SHABD YOGA 173

There is an essential and indivisible relationship between God and the God-man, for he serves as a human pole at which the God-power plays its part and helps in the regeneration of the jivas. It is needless to distinguish between the magnet and the magnetized field and it is therefore said:

> *Devotion to the Satguru is devotion to the Lord,*
> *Satguru secures salvation by giving contact with*
> *Naam (the God-power).*

Uncovetous of worldly riches, he may seem poor, but he is rich in God's Infinitude and, once the mortal coils have been cast off, he is reabsorbed into the still center, subject to no limitations. What gives him his unique preeminence is precisely this spiritual at-one-ment with the Absolute, and to judge him on the human level is to fail to understand him. Rumi has well said, "Never take a God-man to be human; for though appearing so, he is yet much more." It is by virtue of the extra-human potential that he becomes the Master. Having merged into Divine Consciousness he, in his human state, becomes Its agent and speaks not in his individual capacity but as the mouthpiece of God:

> *His hand is the hand of God*
> *And the power of the Lord works through him.*
> RUMI

> *O! my friend, I speak nothing from myself,*
> *I only utter what the Beloved puts into my mouth.*
> GURU NANAK

> *I do nothing of myself; but as my Father hath*
> *taught me, I speak these things.*
> ST. JOHN

The Master being what he is, it is not surprising that he should be held so high. Being an instrument of the Divine, to praise him is only another way of praising God, and to extol him above God is not to set up an opposition between the finite and the Infinite but to assert that from the human standpoint, the aspect of God which bends down toward man to raise him to Itself (i.e., the centripetal), is higher than that which merely allows him to run his ways in the world of relativity from birth to birth (i.e., the centrifugal), even though both at the supra-human level are seen to be one and indivisible.

A system in which the teacher is so central to every aspect of the student's outer and inner discipline and progress and without whose instruction and guidance nothing could be done, must lay great emphasis on the principle of Grace, and mystic literature is not wanting in stressing and underlining this aspect. But if from one angle it is the Master who bestows everything upon the disciple, it must not be forgotten that in doing this he is only repaying a debt he owes to his own Guru, for the gift he bestows is the gift he himself received when he was at the stage of a disciple, and so he usually never claims anything for himself but attributes his power to the grace of his own teacher. Besides, from another angle, everything is in the disciple himself and the Master does not add anything from outside. It is only when the gardener waters and tends the seed that it bursts into life, yet the secret of life is in the seed itself and the gardener can do no more than provide the conditions for its fructification. Such indeed is the function of the Guru.

An ancient Indian parable vividly brings out this aspect of Master-disciple relationship. It relates that once a shepherd trapped a lion's cub and reared him with the rest of his flock. The cub, judging himself by those he saw around him, lived and moved like the sheep and lambs, content with the grass they nibbled and with the weak bleats they emitted. And so time sped on until, one day, another lion saw the growing cub grazing with the rest of the flock. He guessed what had happened and pitying the cub's plight, he went up to him, drew him to the side of a quiet stream, made him behold his reflection and the lion's own and, turning back, let forth a mighty roar. The cub, now understanding his true nature, did likewise and his erstwhile companions fled before him. He was at last free to enjoy his rightful place and thenceforward roamed about as a king of the forest.

The Master is indeed such a lion. He comes to stir up the soul from its slumber and, presenting it with a mirror, makes it behold its own innate glory of which, without his touch, it would continue unaware. However, were it not itself of the essence of life, nothing could raise it to spiritual consciousness. The Guru is but a lighted candle that lights the unlit ones. The fuel is there, the wick is there, he only gives the gift of flame without any loss to himself. Like touches like, the spark passes between and that which lay dark is illumined and that which was dead springs into life. As with the lighted candle, whose privilege lies not in its being an individual candle but in its being the seat of the unindividual flame that is neither of this candle nor of that but of the very essence of all fire, so too with the true Master. He is a Master not by virtue of his being an individual master like anyone else, but he is a Master carrying in him the Universal Light of God. Again, just as only a candle that is still burning can light other candles—not one that is already burnt out—so only a living Master can give the quickening touch that is needed, not one who has already departed from this world. Those that are gone were great indeed and worthy of all respect, but they were preeminently for their own time, and the task they accomplished for those around them must, for us, be performed by one who lives and moves in our midst. Their memory is a sacred treasure, a perennial source of inspiration, but the one thing their remembrance teaches is to seek for ourselves in the world of the living that which they themselves were. Only the kiss of a living Prince (Master) could bring the slumbering Princess (Soul) back to life and only the touch of a breathing Beauty could restore the Beast to his native pristine glory.

Where the guidance of a competent living Master is such a prime necessity, the task of finding and recognizing such a genuine soul assumes paramount importance. There is no dearth of false prophets and of wolves in sheep's clothing. The very term *Satguru,* or true Master, implies the existence of its opposite, and it is the false that meet our gaze at every turn. However difficult it may be to find a God-man (for such beings are rare, unobtrusive in their humility and reluctant to declare themselves by spectacular miracles or court the public limelight), it is nevertheless not impossible to single him out from the rest. He is a living embodiment of what he teaches, and though appearing poor, he is rich in his poverty:

> *We may seem beggars, but our actions are more*
> *than royal.*

SHAMAS TABREZ

He is unattached to worldly objects and is never covetous. He gives his teachings and instructions as a free gift of nature, never seeking anything in return, maintaining himself by his own labors and never living on the offerings of others:

> *Bow not before one who calls himself a Master, yet*
> *lives on the charity of others.*
> *He alone is of the true path who earns his own liveli-*
> *hood and befriends the needy.*

GURU RAM DAS

Further, a genuine Master-soul never sets up any contradictions in our minds; all the distinctions between faith and faith, creed and creed, vanish at his touch, and the unity of inner experience embodied in the various scriptures stands clearly revealed:

> *It is only the jeweller's eye that at a glance can tell the ruby.*

BHAI NAND LAL

The one recurrent theme of such a Master's teaching is that in spite of all the outward distinctions that confuse and confound us, the inner spiritual essence of all religious teachings is the same. Hence the Masters come not to propagate new creeds or dogmas but to fulfill the existing Law:

> *O Nanak, know him to be a perfect Master who unites all in one fold.*

GURU NANAK

If he tries to convert, it is not the outward name and form that he seeks, but the baptism of the spirit within. For him, the inner life is a science that is open to men of all creeds and nations, and whosoever shall take up its discipline, to him shall all things be added.

Thus it is the inner message that is ever paramount in the teachings of a real Master. He can best interpret the true import of the scriptures but he speaks not as one who is learned in such matters but as one who has himself experienced what such writings record. He may use the scriptures to convince his listeners that what he teaches is the most ancient truth, yet he himself is never subject to them and his message moves above the merely intellectual level; it is inspired by the vividness and intensity of direct first-hand experience. "How can we agree," said Kabir to the theoretical pandits, "when I speak from inner experience and you only from bookish learning." He makes the seeker turn always inward, telling him of the rich treasures within:

Dost thou reckon thyself a puny form,
When within thee the Universe is folded?

ALI

The kingdom of God cometh not with observation,
The kingdom of God is within you.

ST. LUKE

Inviting and persuading him to undertake the discipline
that unlocks this treasure he says:

Cleanse thou the rheum from thy head
And breathe the light of God instead.

RUMI

And this discipline, if he be indeed a perfect teacher, will
focus itself not on Hatha Yoga or other such extreme practices, but on transcendental hearing and seeing accompanied
by a steady outer purification of one's thoughts and deeds by
means of moderation and introspective self-criticism, rather
than by torture, austerity or asceticism. But the most important and least fallible sign of the Satguru is that his teachings
will not only always be centered on this inner science, but at
the time of initiation, he will be able to give the disciple a
definite experience—be it ever so rudimentary—of the Light
and Sound within and, when the disciple has learned to rise
above body-consciousness, his Radiant Form will appear unsought to guide him onward on the long journey.

The wondrous and luminous form of the Master
only a true Master can make manifest to the spirit.

GURU NANAK

He is a Guru in vain who cannot turn the darkness (*gu*)
into light (*ruh*). And Nanak has said, "I will not take my
Master at his word until I see with mine own eyes." If he is
a genuine teacher, he will never promise salvation that comes

only after death. Accordingly, to him it is always a matter of now and here. One who has not attained liberation in life, cannot hope to achieve it after death. Jesus too always urged his disciples to master the art of dying daily. A Master will further maintain that spirituality is a science, albeit a subjective one, and that every individual can and must verify its truth in the laboratory of his own body, provided he can create the requisite condition, which is one-pointed concentration. Life is one continuous process which knows no end, though it may assume different aspects at different levels of existence. As one passes helplessly from one plane to another, he is supposed to have died at the plane quitted by the soul; for we have yet no knowledge and much less experience of the life on other planes, where one is led by the propelling force of karmic vibrations. It is from this bondage and forced comings and goings that the Master prepares the way to liberation in this very life, by connecting a jiva to the eternal lifelines pervading endlessly through the creation, and gives one an actual foretaste of the higher spiritual regions, provided one is prepared to forsake the flesh for the spirit. "Learn to die, that you may begin to live," exhorted the Master Christian. Blessed is the man who daily prepares himself to die.

Those in whom the eternal Word speaks are delivered from uncertainty, and it is indeed the Master's job to make this Word audible in man.

> O Nanak! snap all the ties of the world,
> Serve the true Master and He shall bestow on thee
> true riches.
>
> GURBANI

He who has such a teacher is blessed indeed, for he has verily made friends with God Himself and found a companion who shall not forsake him even to the end of the earth, in this life or after death, and who shall not cease to guide him until he reaches his final destination and becomes as great and infinite as himself.

> *A philosopher's stone at best may turn base metal into gold,*
> *But glory to the Master who can transform the disciple into his own celestial mould.*

Whatever one's problems, there is peace and solace in his company, and association with him gives strength and stimulates inner effort; hence the pressing need for Satsang (association with the True One), for those who have not yet learned to commune with him on the inner planes.

A seeker must certainly be critical and discriminating in his search for a perfect Master, but having succeeded in finding one (and he who is a genuine seeker will never fail, such is the Divine decree), what will be the nature of his relationship to him? Will he continue to be critical of what he is told and observes? Will he continue to test every act of his teacher with the microscope of his discrimination? To maintain such an attitude even after having initially ascertained the genuineness of the Perfect One is to fail to appreciate his greatness and rightly respond to it. To meet such a soul is to meet one infinitely greater than oneself, and to know him to be one with God is to be humbled and full of awe. To judge him by one's limited faculties is to attempt to hold the ocean in a test-tube, for he is moved by reasons that we can never comprehend.

He who can appreciate the blessing of being taken into the fold of the Satguru or the *murshid-i-kamil,* will forever sing of his Grace, beauty and perfect love:

> *If the beautiful One were to take my wandering soul under his wing, I would sacrifice all empires for the lovely mole on his face.*

> HAFIZ

He will never question the actions of his Master, even if he fails to understand them, for he knows that even:

> *If Khizr did wreck the vessel on the sea*
> *Yet in this wrong there are a thousand rights.*

RUMI

He will have to develop the faith of a child who, having trusted himself to a loving hand, moves as directed, never questioning anything:

> *. . . whosoever shall not receive the Kingdom of*
> *God as a little child shall in no wise enter therein.*

ST. LUKE

> *Even if he asks thee to dye the seat of worship with*
> *wine, be not scandalized, but do it,*
> *For He who is thy Guide knows well the journey and*
> *its stages.*

RUMI

The cryptic words of the God-man very often baffle human understanding. His behests, at times, may apparently sound contrary to the scriptural texts or ethical injunctions, but in reality they are not. One should follow them in full faith, and in due time their true significance will be revealed.

And like the child's should be the devotee's love, full of humility and simplicity. The purity of its flame alone shall burn away the dross of the world:

> *Kindle the fire of love and burn all things,*
> *Then set thy foot unto the land of the lovers.*

BAHA'U'LLAH

Weld into one the vessel, which is now fragmented into a thousand parts, so that it may be fit to contain the light of God. It is the link between the seeker and his Friend and through Him, between the seeker and the Absolute. How can

one love the Nameless and Formless but through Him, who is
His true embodiment, for as the Lord revealed to Mohammed:

> *I dwell neither high nor low, neither in the sky nor*
> *on the earth, nor even in paradise,*
> *O beloved, believe me, strange as it may seem,*
> *I dwell in the heart of the faithful and it is there*
> *that I may be found.*
>
> RUMI

On this mystic path reasoning is the help, but reasoning
is also the hindrance. Love alone can bridge the gulf, span
the chasm, and knit the finite to the Infinite, the mortal to the
Immortal, the relative to the Absolute. Such love is not of this
world or of this flesh. It is the call of soul unto soul, of like
unto like, the purgatory and the paradise. Who shall describe
its ecstasy?

> *Speak not of Leila's or of Majnun's woe*
> *Thy love hath put to naught the loves of long ago.*
>
> SAADI

> *Live free of love for its very peace is anguish.*
>
> ARABIAN POEM

> *A million speak of love, yet how few know,*
> *True love is not to lose remembrance even for an*
> *instant.*
>
> KABIR

Indeed, it is the quality of ceaseless remembrance that is of
the essence of love. He who remembers in such fashion must
needs to live in perpetual remembrance of his Beloved's commandments and in perpetual obedience. Such love burns in
its fire the dross of the ego; the little self is forgotten and the
lover surrenders his individuality at the altar of his Beloved:

If thou wouldst journey on the road of love,
First learn to humble thyself unto dust.

ANSARI OF HERAT

Love grows not in the field and is not sold in the
market,
Whosoever would have it, whether king or beggar,
must pay with his life.
Carry your head upon your palm as an offering,
If you would step into the Wonderland of love.

KABIR

Again:

Accursed be the life wherein one finds not love for
the Lord;
Give your heart to His servant for He shall take you
to Him.

Such self-surrender is only a prelude to the inheriting of a larger and purer Self than we otherwise know, for such is the potency of its magic that whosoever shall knock at its door shall be transformed into its own color:

A lover becomes the Beloved — such is the alchemy
of his love;
God Himself is jealous of such a Beloved.

DADU

Calling on Ranjha, I myself become one with him.

BULLEH SHAH

It is of such a love that Lord Krishna spoke in the Gita, and of such a love that St. Paul preached to his listeners:

I am crucified with Christ; nevertheless I live; yet
not I, but Christ liveth in me: and the life which I
now live in the flesh I live by the faith of the Son of
God, who loved me, and gave himself for me.

ST. PAUL

It is of this that the Sufis speak when they talk of *fana-fil-sheikh* (annihilation in the Master):

> *The vast expanse of myself is so filled to overflowing with the fragrance of the Lord that the very thought of myself has completely vanished.*

It is of this that the Christian mystics declare when they stress the necessity of "Death in Christ." Without such self-surrender, learning by itself can be of little avail:

> *Learning is only a child of the scriptures,*
> *It is love that is their mother.*
>
> PERSIAN POEM

> *The world is lost in reading scriptures, yet never comes to knowledge,*
> *But one who knows a jot of love, to him all is revealed.*
>
> KABIR

Such love alone is the key to the inner kingdom:

> *He that loveth not knoweth not God, for God is love.*
>
> ST. JOHN

> *The secret of God's mysteries is love.*
>
> RUMI

> *By love may He be gotten and holden, but by thought never.*
>
> THE CLOUD OF UNKNOWING

> *Verily, verily I say unto thee, that only they that have loved have reached the Lord.*
>
> GOBIND SINGH

And we have known and believed the love that God
hath to us. God is love; and he that dwelleth in love
dwelleth in God, and God in him.

ST. JOHN

We love him, because he first loved us.

ST. JOHN

This relationship of love between the Satguru and his shish-
ya, the Godman and his disciple, covers many phases and
many developments. It begins with respect for one knowing
more than oneself. As the disciple begins to appreciate the
Master's disinterested solicitude for his welfare and progress,
his feelings begin to soften with the dew of love and he begins
to develop faith, obedience and reverence. With greater obedience and faith comes greater effort, and with greater effort
comes greater affection from the Master. Effort and grace go
hand in hand and each in turn helps in development of the
other. Like the mother's love for her children is the love of
the divine shepherd for his flock. It does not discriminate
between the deserving and the undeserving but like the mother, the depths and treasures of his love are unlocked only to
those who respond and return his love:

He is with all alike, yet each gets his share according
to his own deserts.

GURU AMAR DAS

With his greater effort and the greater grace from the
Master, the disciple makes increased headway in his inner
sadhnas, leading finally to complete transcendence of bodily
consciousness. When this transcendence has been achieved, he
beholds his Guru waiting in his Radiant Form to receive and
guide his spirit on the inner planes. Now, for the first time, he
beholds him in his true glory, and realizes the unfathomable
dimensions of his greatness. Henceforth he knows him to be

more than human and his heart overflows with songs of praise and humble devotion. The higher he ascends in his spiritual journey, the more insistent is he in his praise, for the more intensely does he realize that he whom he once took to be a friend, is not merely a friend but God Himself come down to raise him up to Himself. This bond of love, with its development by degrees, becomes the mirror of his inward progress, moving as it does, from the finite to the Infinite:

Love begins in the flesh and ends in the spirit.

ST. BERNARD

At its initial phase, it may find analogies in earthly love, that between the parent and the child, friend and friend, lover and beloved, teacher and pupil, but once it has reached the point where the disciple discovers his teacher in his luminous glory within himself, all analogies are shattered and all comparisons forever left behind; all that remains is a gesture, and then silence:

Let us write some other way
Love's secrets — better so.
Leave blood and noise and all of these
And speak no more of Shamas Tabrez.

RUMI

CHAPTER SIX

The Essence of Religion

IN THE preceding chapter, we sketched the main outlines
of the Surat Shabd Yoga and briefly examined its outstanding features. We saw how it posits that God, when He
projected himself into manifestation, took form as the Word,
Naam, Shabd, Udgit, Kalma, Saut or Sraosha, and that these
terms refer not to abstract concepts of Divine Will or Reason
but to something more; a spiritual stream of celestial harmony
radiant with effulgence. This stream is at the center of all
creation, bringing into being its various planes, vitalizing and
sustaining them. He, who under the guidance of one who has
himself mastered the Way, can contact this current within,
can transcend the physical world and steadily rise above all
planes of relativity and, when he becomes one with It, reach
back into Its very source thus escaping from the realms of
limitation to that of Infinite Consciousness and Absolute
Being.

To indicate that these teachings are not restricted to any
one people or any one age but have a universal applicability,
every important aspect was briefly illustrated from the sayings
of mystics drawn from various religious traditions: Indian,
Islamic and Christian. However, these sayings are only by
way of illustrative references. If the tenets of the Surat Shabd
Yoga are indeed universal, if they really point to absolute truth
and are based not on dogma but on "facts," albeit of a supra-
physical nature, but facts which can be verified by anyone

187

who is ready to undergo the discipline demanded for their
study, then the inquiring seeker would surely assert that these
tenets should, in some form or the other, be at the heart of
all great religions, and he would desire a more systematic
demonstration of this than has been possible in the foregoing
account of the Surat Shabd Yoga. A comprehensive and detailed treatment of this subject is beyond the scope of this book,
and at best we can only suggest some fruitful lines of enquiry,
which those desiring to go further may pursue. Besides, it
is a recurrent theme of all great Masters, that though their
teachings are universal in nature and may be verified from
the extensive scriptural literature* of the world, yet to confine
oneself merely to learned interpretation is to miss completely
the true import of their teachings. All that the seeker needs to
do is to ascertain from past records that what he is being told
is the most ancient of truths, so that he may take up the
discipline required with full faith and without reservation.
Final verification must be a matter of direct and first-hand
inner experience and not one of bookish learning, which, when
carried beyond its proper limit and made an end in itself,
defeats its purpose and becomes a serious distraction from the
goal.

I. Ancient Religious Thought:
Indian, Chinese and Iranian

Hinduism

The Hindu religion is a vast ocean of religious thought,
springing as it does from the earliest times, long before the
dawn of history, and comprises in its multi-colored texture
shade after shade, an endless variety of design and pattern as
it grew in the human mind; from animism to Nature wor-

*For more details, the reader is invited to the book *Naam or Word* by
the same author.

ship, from powers of Nature in the abstract to personified and concretized natural forms, from gods and goddesses to the one Supreme God, first personal, and then impersonal; from form to formless. The Hindu Pantheon offers a view of a vast and mighty host to the curious inquirer who pierces into the mists of the hoary past.

Heliolatry, the worship of *Helios* or the Sun, was a common practice with the people of the world. Sol or Sun has ever been an object of great veneration for man and has been adored and worshiped all the world over from time immemorial. The ancient Greeks and the Romans built temples to Apollo or Phoebus as they termed the Sun-god in their own time. In all their temples, the image or representation of the Sun-god occupied an important place in their hierarchy. There is a famous Sun-temple in Konark, in South India, and in the historic town of Mooltan or the land of the Sun, in the North. In addition, *Jog-maya* or *Jot-maya* temples dot the whole Indian subcontinent.

The ancient Greeks also spoke of *Shabd*. It is written of Socrates that he heard within him a peculiar sound which pulled him irresistibly into higher spiritual realms. Pythagoras also talked of Shabd, for he described God as "Supreme Music of the nature of Harmonies." God was to him, "Absolute Truth, clothed in light." When he commanded an eagle to fly down to him and a bear to stop ravaging Apulia, the wondering multitude inquired of him the source from where such powers came to him. He replied that he owed it all to the "Science of Light."

Again, in the Greek language we have the mystical word *Logos*. It comes from the root *lego* which means to speak and from it we have the common terms, monologue, dialogue, prologue, epilogue and so on. The Logos means and stands for the "Word" or "Reason." The term *Logos* also occurs in both Hebrew and Christian philosophy and theology and is used, in its mystic sense, by the Hellenistic and Neo-platonist philosophers. The Christians use it to denote the second person of the Trinity.

The ancients in the West inherited this concept from their ancestors who, thousands of years before the Christian era, had come to acquire a great love and adoration for *Surya* which they regarded as the be-all and the end-all of all human endeavors in their search for the mighty power of God, and as a visible representation to this earth. They carried this notion along with them wherever they went, Eastward or Westward, and composed hymns and chanted psalms in praise of the glorious orb, the source of all life on this solar planet. Those who settled in Iran (Persia) and came subsequently to be known as Parsees, still worship the great deity in yet another form—fire—which they keep burning all the time in their temples as symbolic of the sacred flame that burnt in the human heart and always sprang heavenward. Ratu Zoroaster, the Iranian prophet of life and light, sang in loving and living faith of the greatness of the God of Light and taught the people to do so.

Agni or fire was a hidden secret with the gods, who guarded this mysterious power very jealously. It was, as the Greek legend goes, stolen by Prometheus and given to man, for which Jupiter, the father god, bound him to eternal torture. In Chapter VI of the Chhandogya Upanishad, it is said to be "the prime element whose creation made possible that of other elements, water, earth," etc.

The second branch of the Aryans which turned eastward into the Indo-Gangetic plain also referred lovingly to *Aditya;* and we have hymns in the Vedas addressed to *Hiranyagarbha, Savitar* and *Usha,* all of which stand for the One life-sustaining power, the Sun. The worshipful Masters of the Vedic age were, one and all, admirers of the purifying and healing attributes of the Sun-god, and so no wonder that we see many hymns in the Vedic literature deifying the sun. In Book X, 121, we find:

> *In the beginning rose Hiranyagarbha, born as the*
> *only lord of all created beings;*
> *He fixed and holdeth up this earth and heaven;*
> *What god shall we adore with our oblation?* . . .
> *What time the mighty water came, containing the*
> *Universal germ, producing Agni,*
> *Thence sprang the God's One Spirit into being:*
> *What god shall we adore with our oblation?*

In another hymn, he is referred to as "the self-radiant wise Aditya."

In Book I, 113, we have a hymn to Dawn and in it occur, inter alia, the following lines:

> *This light is come, amid all lights the fairest; born is*
> *the brilliant, far-extending brightness.*
> *Night, sent away for Savitar's uprising, hath yielded*
> *up a birthplace, for the morning . . .*
> *Arise! the breath, the life, again hath reached us:*
> *darkness hath passed away, and light approacheth.*
> *She for the sun hath left a path to travel; we have*
> *arrived where men prolong existence.*

All this could be taken on the literal plane as little more than Nature-worship, an adoration of the sun, understandable among a people dependent upon agriculture for their existence. But ancient Indian literature has an elusive quality. It seems to teach us at one level, and when we have adjusted ourselves to it, it suddenly shifts us to another. He who can follow its subtleties finds in it a richness rarely to be met elsewhere. There is multiplicity of meanings, ranging from the physical to the cosmic and the spiritual, and from the literal to the symbolic and esoteric, which challenge us at multiple levels of experience and offer us worthwhile rewards. Thus, when we begin studying these frequent references to the sun, we begin to see that the "sun" referred to is not always the center of our physical Universe, which we initially took it to be. Thus, in the Isha Upanishad, we are told:

> *The door of the True One is covered with a golden disk.*
> *Open that, O Pushan, that we may see the nature of the True One.*

After recounting such statements, when we read of Brahman or the Supreme One, as being *Jyotisvat,* full of light, and *Prakashvat,* endowed with splendor, we begin to discover in such terms an esoteric significance we earlier overlooked. This comes to a head when we read the *Gayatri,* the tenth mantra of the sixteenth sutra in the third mandala of the Rig Veda:

> *Muttering the sacred syllable "Aum" rise above the three regions,*
> *And turn thy attention to the All-Absorbing Sun within.*
> *Accepting its influence be thou absorbed in the Sun,*
> *And it shall in its own likeness make thee All-Luminous.*

This mantra is considered the most sacred, the *mool mantra* among the Vedic texts, and is taught for recitation among Hindus from an early age. Here, the inner spiritual meaning of the "Sun" becomes abundantly clear. The object of veneration is not that which provides us with light in the outside world but it is a principle that transcends the three planes of existence, the physical, the astral and the causal, and is the source of inner illumination. This principle is referred to as *Aum,* a term whose three letters suggest the three phases of human experience: "A" referring to the waking state (*jag-rat*), "U" the dream state (*swapna*) and "M" the deep sleep state (*sushupti*). The ultimate reality includes all three planes, and the three phases of human experience, yet goes beyond them. The silence that follows each recitation of the word *Aum* suggests the state of Turiya or Absolute Being, which is the indescribable source and end of everything. It is the Brahman, the All-transcending One, whose prime attribute is effulgence, but who is in himself even beyond this effulgence. Hence the mantra in its original Rig Veda form has another line added to it, which is given out only to sanyasins and chosen disciples—*Paro Raj-asal Savad Aum*: He who transcends the effulgence is this Aum.

The Gayatri not only clarifies the routine implications of the references to the sun, abundant in the Vedas, but it also highlights another recurring theme in Hindu thought. Its wide imagery and popularity bring us to the question of mantras and their place in Indian religious practice. The mantras or verbal formulae in Sanskrit verse or prose are classified into two types: those that are meant simply for recitation and need not be understood, and those that are divine invocations, whose import must be known in order to enable the devotee to keep his attention focused on the divine object. The various mantras each have their individual benefits. There are those whose mastery or *siddhi* gives one contact with magical powers of a lower order (*tamsic*); there are others that bestow strength and courage and power (*rajsic*); and finally those whose sole object is spiritual upliftment (*satvic*). Among the last, as we have already seen, the Gayatri is the most venerated.

The mode of mantras, since time immemorial, stresses the spiritual importance of Sound. If the chanting of certain verbal formulae brings magical potential or assists spiritual advancement, then there must be latent in Sound itself an esoteric power. This is why Vak Devi, the goddess of speech, was held in high esteem. Each word has its unique character and place, but of all words *Aum* is the most sacred. We have already examined some of its symbolic meanings. To these we may add still others. It is not only a term that connotes the qualities of the Absolute Brahman, but one that also denotes Brahman Himself. In the Rig Veda, we have:

> *Prajapati vai idam agref aseet*
> *Tasya vag dvitya aseet,*
> *Vag vai parmam Brahma.*

("In the beginning was Prajapati, the Brahman, with whom was the Word and the Word was verily the Supreme Brahman.") This text remarkably parallels the opening of the Gospel according to St. John:

> *In the beginning was the Word, and the Word was*
> *with God and the Word was God.*

Thus *Aum* becomes Brahman as manifesting Itself in the Word, and in the Taittriya Upanishad, It is referred to as the "Sheath of Brahman," as something which takes Its life from Brahman and contains Him. This aspect is made even clearer in the Sam Veda:

> *Brahman is at once Shabd and Ashabd both,*
> *And Brahman alone vibrates in space.*

In other words, the Absolute One is not only inner effulgence but also beyond it, as suggested in the Gayatri. He is with the Word, the Shabd or *Aum,* yet beyond It. Both Sound and Light are in fact referred to as His prime manifestations. The Gayatri recommends that while concentrating on the Divine Word *Aum,* we fix our attention upon the inner Sun, while in the Chhandogya Upanishad, we are told that *Naad,* or the divine music, springs from the Universal Sun (of Brahmand), a secret that was given by Angris Rishi to

Krishna, the darling son of Devki (III:17-6 and 93). It was this mystic insight to be found in the *srutis,* the scriptures revealed through inner hearing, that led to the development of what came to be called the *Sphota-vada* or the philosophy of the Word. The teachers of this path preached that the Absolute was Wordless, imageless, indescribable and unconditioned. When He came into manifestation, He projected Himself as the *Sphota* or the Word, radiant with Light and vibrating with indescribable Music. The seeker wishing to transcend the relative plane to the Eternal and Unchanging must contact the Sphota or the Word Power through which he can rise to the Brahman who is beyond Shabd or Sphota. The Path of God-realization is certainly not easy. It is difficult to have access to, difficult to cognize, difficult to abide by and difficult to cross; yet it is the only possible Way, for one who is true to his Guru and His cause.

Such indeed are the truths that were taught and practiced by the forest sages of ancient India. But how much of them has survived since then? For the most part we find rituals such as the blowing of conches, ringing of bells, waving of lights, and the worship of the sun. These bear testimony to the mysteries within, but how few are conscious of their real significance? In spite of Lord Krishna's powerful and lasting influence which brought the best of the Vedantic teachings to the heart of the common man, religion in India as elsewhere has tended to degenerate into mere caste and ceremony. The light and music outside are worshiped, but the flaming and sounding Word within, toward which they point, goes unheeded; "the light crieth in the darkness and the darkness comprehendeth it not."

Buddhism

The teachings of Buddha represent in many ways a reaction against the religious traditions, some distorted, of the

Vedas, and yet they confirm many of the basic tenets that we have already examined. The life of Buddha himself has become a legend embodying in a vivid and striking way, man's need to turn from the phenomenal, outer world, to the noumenal, inner one. With his royal lineage and with everything that could make life happy at home, Buddha's going out of the palace into the wilderness as a mendicant in quest of Truth was an unprecedented sacrifice. It indeed was a heroic endeavor on his part to wander for six long years, and to resort to all sorts of austerities and physical sufferings, reducing himself to a bare skeleton, and this compels deep and abiding admiration and adoration. But neither the life of luxury at home nor of tapas in the jungles could help him solve the problem of the misery, distress, sickness and death, which he had witnessed as the common lot of man's life in the physical world. It was a momentous decision of his to forsake the ascetic life as he had done the one of luxury before. Seated under the Bodhi tree in Gaya, in calm contemplation, he gave himself up to the divine influence that operates of itself and by itself when one resigns his self completely to the holiest and the highest in Nature, when suddenly there flashed upon his inward eye the much sought solution to the most baffling problem of life, in a seriated chain of cause and effect: (1) the undeniable fact of suffering, (2) the cause of suffering, (3) the possibility of removing suffering, and lastly, (4) the path that leads to freedom from suffering. This was the Path of the Golden Mean, between self-indulgence and self-mortification, both of which were equally painful and unprofitable in the search after truth. Hence it was given the name of the Middle Path, consisting of righteousness in the eightfold aspects of life, which have already been described in the earlier part of this book.

This, in brief, was the purport of the Master's first sermon at Sarnath, delivered to the first five *Bhikkus*. The simple and

direct teachings, free from sophistications of the priestly order
—the Brahmins—who had made rites and rituals as the be-all
and end-all of man's salvation, had a tremendous influence on
the people as a whole. No wonder then that the new faith had
a large number of converts from the ruling chiefs down to the
laymen, who eagerly took to the yellow robe.

This is the outer aspect as in all other religions of the world
before and after Buddha's time, and it worked well with the
masses, for it gave them a clear perspective of life and life's
way. The intricate Vedic problems, the Vedic Pantheon and
the Vedic mode of worship were bypassed in a single sweep,
and the people were asked to evolve and elevate their conduct
and everything else would follow of itself. This was, in a way,
the strict observance of yamas and niyamas that go to make
for Sadachar (right conduct), the first and foremost step in
the right direction.

It does not mean that Buddha denied the existence either
of God, or of the steps leading up to Him on the spiritual
path. A mere public non-affirmation of something of higher
value and vital interest far ahead of his time and which the
common man was not yet prepared and ready to accept does
not mean the negation of the same. The higher Path was of
course left for the chosen few and kept for the elect, who
were worthy of the mystical teaching relating to transcendental hearing, as we read in the *Surangama Sutra,* wherein
are described the spiritual experiences of the highest *Bodhis-
atvas* and *Mahasatvas* and great *Arhats,* like Maha Kasyapa,
Sariputra, Samant Bhadra, Metaluniputra, Maudgalyana,
Akshobya, Vejuria, Maitreya, Mahasthema-Prapta and others. All of them in their accounts testify, in one form or
another, to the purple-golden brightness, the infinitude of
pure mind-essence, the transcendental perception, the transcendental and intrinsic hearing experienced by the inner mind,
leading to the indescribable and mysterious Sound of Dharma

like the roar of a lion or the beating of drums; the penetrating power of the element of fire, making the intuitive insight luminously clear and enabling them to view all the Deva realms and finally the Buddha-land of Immovability, laying bare to the core the very heart of balanced and rhythmic ethereal vibrations. They also speak of the "Supreme, wonderful and perfect Samadhi of Transcendental Consciousness" called the "Diamond Samadhi," that is attainable by means of "Intrinsic Hearing," when the mind, freed from mental contaminations, loses itself into the "Divine Stream."

After listening to the various personages, Manjusri, the prince of Dharma, laid great stress on attaining "the supreme purity of mind-essence and its intrinsic brightness shining spontaneously in all directions," and exhorted the Great Assembly "to reverse the outward perception of hearing and to listen inwardly to the perfectly unified and intrinsic Sound of the mind-essence." He then summed up the subject in the following memorable words:

> This is the only way to Nirvana, and it has been followed by all the Tathagatas of the past. Moreover, it is for all the Bodhisatvas and Mahasatvas of the present and for all in the future if they are to hope for perfect enlightenment. Not only did Avalokiteswara attain perfect enlightenment in long ages past by this Golden Way, but in the present, I also, am one of them . . . I bear testimony that the means employed by Avalokiteswara is the most expedient means for all.*

Again, the contemplators in the Hinayana school of Buddhism were also called *Shravaks* which means "hearers," i.e., hearers of the inner Sound-principle.

But after the passing away of the Lord, the secret teachings given by him to the chosen few gradually disappeared, and

* For a fuller account in this connection, see the section "Evidence from Various Religions" in *Naam or Word* by the same author.

Buddhism like all other religions after having served the great need of the hour, now remains just a collection of dogmas and beliefs and offers little solace to the seekers after Truth, which comes only from a Truth-realized soul, a real saint with spiritual attainment and inner experience of the Reality.

Taoism

Turning to China, we find the best in Buddhist thought passing into the religious traditions of the Chinese. But along with this, we may note the message taught on his own by Lao Tze, the father of Chinese Mysticism (*Hsuanchiao*) or Taoism. The term *Tao* meaning "road" or way, denotes the hidden "principle of the universe."

Lao Tze speaks of Tao as "Absolute Tao" which is the "Essence" and "Quintessence" (the spiritual truth) quite apart from and yet immanent in its manifestations. Just as Indian mystics had distinguished between the *Aum* that we chant and the *Aum* that is the Indescribable, Inexpressible, Wordless Word, so too Lao Tze tells us:

The Tao that can be told of
Is not the Absolute Tao;
The names that can be given
Are not Absolute Names.

Of the character of Tao, it is further said:

Tao is all-pervading
And Its use is inexhaustible!
Fathomless!
Like the fountainhead of all things.

Again:

The Great Tao flows everywhere,
(Like a flood) It may go left or right.
The myriad things derive their life from It,
And It does not deny them.

And again:

> *The Tao never does,*
> *Yet through It everything is done.*

In Book II, dealing with the application of Tao, is given the Principle of Reversion:

> *Reversion is the action of Tao,*
> *Gentleness is the function of Tao,*
> *The things of this world come from Being,*
> *And Being comes from Non-Being.*

Tao is the source of all knowledge:

> *Without stepping outside one's door,*
> *One knows what is happening in the world.*
> *Without looking out of one's window,*
> *One can see the Tao of Heaven.*
> *The further one possesses knowledge,*
> *The less one knows.*
> *Therefore the sage knows without running about,*
> *Understands without seeing,*
> *Accomplishes without doing.*

The Grand Harmony of Tao, the mysterious secret of the universe, becomes manifest when:

> *When the mystic virtue becomes clear, far-reaching,*
> *And things revert back (to their source),*
> *Then and then only emerges the Grand Harmony.*

Of his own teachings (as of the great sages), he said:

> *My teachings are very easy to understand and very*
> *easy to practice,*
> *But no one can understand them and none can prac-*
> *tice them.*
> *In my words there is a principle,*

In the affairs of man there is system,
Because they know not these
They also know me not.
Since there are few that know me,
Therefore I am distinguished.
Therefore the sage wears a coarse cloth,
But carries jade within his bosom.

And finally, speaking of the Way to Heaven, he says:

True words are not fine sounding,
Fine-sounding words are not true.
A good man does not argue;
He who argues is not a good man.
The wise one does not know many things;
He who knows many things is not wise.
The sage does not accumulate (for himself).
He lives for other people,
And grows richer in himself;
He gives to other people,
And has greater abundance.
The Tao of Heaven
Blesses, but does not harm.
The way of the sage
Accomplishes, but does not contend.

From the above, it would be clear that Tao is the Way; the Way to Reality, the ineffable and transcendent, the very ground of all existence, the womb from which all life comes into being. It comes only through the cultivation of stillness, or ridding the mind of the mind-stuff, a stillness which but a few can practice, enjoy and radiate to others. The process of approach to inwardness lies through reversion and purification of the spirit by putting the "self" aside. "Bide in silence, and the radiance of the spirit shall come and make its home." It is by the alert watch-and-wait method that the mind becomes blank and still. It is to such a mind, that Nature yields her secret. *We Wei* or "Creative Quietude," which comprises and connotes at once "supreme activity" and "supreme relaxation," is vitally necessary for the realization of Tao. It is "life lived beyond tension," that acts as a magic spell. Tao works without working and can never be learned and so "a sensible man prefers the inner to the outer eye." The Way to Tao is ever in concord with nature and comes by a drive toward simplicity. It is a way of life to be lived that brings in the all-embracing continuity of Tao.

But now, Taoism without Lao Tze has lost its original deep meaning and has acquired a secondary sense, denoting just the Way of the Universe, or the Way according to which an individual may order his life, and it is difficult to see how far one can by himself come to Tao by ordering his life without a Master-soul to put him on the Path.

Zoroastrianism

What the Hindus refer to as *Aum, Naad, Shabd,* the Buddhists describe as the Lion roar of Dharma, and Lao Tze as Tao, Ratu Zarathustra, the ancient Persian sage, speaks of as *Sraosha,* or that which is heard:

> *I cause to invoke that Divine Sraosha (i.e. the Word) which is the greatest of all divine gifts for spiritual succour.*
>
> Ha 33:35

> *The Creative Verbum;*
> *Assimilating one's unfolding self with*
> *His all-pervading Reality,*
> *The Omniscient, Self-existent Life-giver has framed*
>   *this mystic Verbum and its melodious rhythm,*
> *With the Divine Order of personal self-sacrifice for*
>   *the Universe, unto the self-sublimating souls.*

*He is that person who, with the Enlightened Superb
Mind can give both these (Mystic Verbum and
Divine Order) through his gracious mouth unto
the mortals.*

Ha 29:7

In Gatha Ushtavaiti, Zoroaster proclaims:

*Thus I reveal the Word which the Most Unfolded
One has taught me,
The Word which is the best for mortals to listen.
Whosoever shall render obedience and steadfast at-
tention unto Me, will attain for one's own self the
All-Embracing Whole Being and immortality;
And through the service of the Holy Divine Spirit
Will realize Mazda Ahura (Godhead).*

Ha 35:8

But today we see only the symbolic fire burning all the time
in the Parsi temples and the Parsi households and the chanting of psalms and hymns regardless of the living Sraosha or
the Creative Verbum, which the noble Iranian himself had
practiced for a number of years on Mt. Alburz and of which
he taught the people, as opposed to the worship of the ancient
gods of Babylon and Nineveh. Bound however to the fiery
symbol of the original Sraosha, it is no wonder that the Parsis
are now known as "fire-worshipers."

Thus we see that each saint or sage, in his time, gave to
the world what he had himself experienced, in a form that
could be easily understood and assimilated by the people in
general. Each one of them is worthy of the highest respect for
his contribution to the sum total of spiritual knowledge that
we have, but a real insight into this knowledge and actual
experience of the spiritual truths cannot be had from the past
Masters, for they cannot now come down to the physical plane
to give a living contact of the holy Word to the people and

establish them in communion with the Holy Spirit, call it by whatever name one may like. This needs the touch of a living Master, who like the past Masters is himself in constant touch with the Word, for all life comes from life as light comes from light.

II. CHRISTIANITY

Jesus Christ was essentially a man of the East, and his teachings are imbued with oriental mysticism. It is even speculated that he spent many of his early years (on which the Gospels are silent) in India, and learned much from the Yogins and the Buddhist monks, in his travels from place to place. He perhaps even started his teachings right in India and may have had a foretaste of persecution from the Brahminical order and the so-called high class social circles for his catholicity of vision, for he did not believe in class barriers and preached the equality of man.*

His contribution to the religious thought of the world may be seen in the emphasis he laid on the need for Universal love, and the Kingdom of God within man; the two cardinal principles known to the ancients long before, but forgotten and ignored in practice.

> *Think not that I am come to destroy the law or the Prophets; I am not come to destroy, but to fulfill.*
>
> MATTHEW 5:17

Let us examine some of the pertinent sayings which reveal that Jesus was conversant with the ancient religious thought and practiced the Path of the Masters of the Audible Life Current, sayings which are often ignored or misconstrued by those studying his teachings today:

* Cf. Nicholas Notovitch, *The Unknown Life of Christ,* Chicago: Indo-American Book Co., 1894.

*The light of the body is the eye; if therefore thine
eye be single, thy whole body shall be full of light.
But if thine eye be evil, thy whole body shall be full
of darkness. If therefore the light that is in thee be
darkness, how great is that darkness.*

MATTHEW 6:22-23

Obviously, "the eye" refers to "the single eye" and the
words "if thine eye be single," mean concentrated awareness
within at the center between and at the back of the eyes.
Again, the words "if thine eye be evil" refer to a state of
mental dispersion without, as opposed to concentration within,
and the result will certainly be "darkness"—darkness born of
ignorance about the true and real values of life, for this is the
greatest ill of the soul.

St. Luke then sounds a note of warning when he says:

*Take heed therefore, that the light which is within
thee be not darkness.*

LUKE 2:35

*What I tell you in darkness, that speak ye in light;
and what ye hear in the ear, that preach ye upon the
housetops.*

MATTHEW 10:27

Here are the words of advice from Jesus to his elect, the
chosen few, viz., to carry to the people openly (in light) the
significance of what they heard in "darkness," that is in secret
meditation, and to tell of the divine melody that they heard
in the ear by means of transcendental hearing.

*But hearing, ye shall hear, and shall not understand;
and seeing ye shall see, and shall not perceive.*

MATTHEW 13:14

The idea conveyed is of the esoteric nature of the spiritual
science which can be experienced in the depths of the soul in

the human laboratory of the body, and cannot be understood on the intellectual level or the level of the senses.

St. Matthew then goes on to explain the matter:

> *For verily I say unto you, that many prophets and righteous men desired to see those things which ye see, and have not seen them; and to hear those things which ye hear; and have not heard them.*

MATTHEW 13:17; LUKE 10:24

In clear and unambiguous words, we have a reference to the inner spiritual experience, a realization of the Kingdom of Light and Harmony, which a real Master like Jesus could make manifest to his disciples.

Like other seers, Jesus gave a mystical experience to his sincere disciples. To the multitude, he always talked in parables, like those of the mustard seed, the fig tree, the ten virgins, etc., with which the Gospels abound.

In a picturesque parable, he explains the sowing of the Word in the hearts of the people, and tells us that the Word sown by the wayside is generally stolen by Satan from the heart; that the Word sown on stony ground takes no roots, endureth for a while and is washed away by the afflictions and persecutions for the Word's sake; that the Word sown among thorns is choked by worldly cares, deceitfulness and lusts of the flesh, and finally, the Word sown on good ground, such as those who hear the Word and receive, brings forth fruit (Mark 4:14-20).

The Path that Jesus taught is one of self-abnegation and of rising above body-consciousness, a process which is tantamount to the experience of death-in-life.

> *Then Jesus said unto his disciples, If any man will come after me, let him deny himself, and take up his cross, and follow me.*
> *For whosoever will save his life shall lose it; and*

*whosoever will lose his life for my sake shall find it.
For what is a man profited, if he shall gain the whole
world and lose his own soul? or what shall a man
give in exchange for his soul?*
                                        MATTHEW 16:24-26

It means one has to sacrifice the outer man, consisting of the
flesh and the carnal mind, for the sake of the Inner man or
soul. In other words, he has to exchange the life of the senses
for the life of the spirit.

Again, the love of God is to be made a ruling passion in life:

*Thou shalt love the Lord thy God with all thy heart,
and with all thy soul, and with all thy mind.*
                                        MATTHEW 22:37

St. Mark goes further and adds, "and with all thy strength"
(Mark 12:30).

*This is the first and great commandment. And the
second is like unto it, Thou shalt love thy neighbor
as thyself. On these two commandments hang all the
law and the prophets.*
MATTHEW 22:37-40; MARK 12:30-31; LUKE 10:27

The principle of love is still further amplified as follows:

*Love your enemies, bless them that curse you, do
good to them that hate you, and pray for them that
despitefully use you, and persecute you.*
                                        MATTHEW 5:44

And why all this?—in order to gain perfection in the likeness
of God:

*Be ye therefore perfect as your Father which is in
heaven is perfect.*
                                        MATTHEW 5:48

In St. Luke, Chapter Three, we are told that "the Word of

God came to John son of Zacharias in the wilderness," and
John while preaching the baptism of repentance for remission
of sins, told the wondering crowd, "I indeed baptize you with
water; but one mightier than I cometh . . . he shall baptize
you with the Holy Ghost and with fire" (Luke 3:2-3, 16)..

We have to mark carefully the words "baptize by the Holy
Ghost" and "fire," for one refers to the heavenly music (the
Holy Word) and the other is symbolic of the heavenly Light,
and these are the twin principles of Sound and Light, the
Primal manifestations of Godhead, or God's Power behind the
entire creation.

The way to the Kingdom of God can be opened unto him
who knows how to "ask" for it, how to "seek" it out and how
to "knock" at the gate. In these three simple words, St. Matthew in Chapter Seven and St. Luke in Chapter Eleven have
summed up what the aspirant has to do. Unfortunately, we
do not yet know where the gate to be knocked at lies. Guru
Nanak also emphatically declares:

O ye blind, ye know not the gate.

About this gate, St. Matthew tells us:

*Enter ye in at the strait gate . . . Because strait is the
gate, and narrow is the way, which leadeth unto life,
and few there be that find it.*

MATTHEW 7:13-14

It is essentially a path of conversion, for no one can enter
into the Kingdom of God unless he is converted and becomes
as a little child (Matthew 18:3), i.e., leaves off his vanities,
becomes meek, pure, simple and innocent like a little child.
St. Luke elaborates on this theme in Chapter 18:15-17, for
when the disciples rebuked them that had brought infants
along, Jesus called them unto him and said, "Suffer little
children to come unto me, and forbid them not, for of such

(like-minded) is the Kingdom of God. Verily I say unto you, whosoever shall not receive the Kingdom of God as a little child shall in no wise enter therein."

In St. John, Chapter One, we come to an elaborate exposition of the teachings of Christ. He begins his gospel with the memorable words, the intrinsic significance of which few have cared to grasp:

> *In the beginning was the Word, and the Word was*
> *with God, and the Word was God.*
> *The same was in the beginning with God.*
> *All things were made by Him; and without Him*
> *was not anything made that was made.*
> *In Him was life; and the life was the light of men.*
> *And the Light shineth in darkness; and the darkness*
> *comprehended it not. . . .*
> *That was the true Light, which lighteth every man*
> *that cometh into the world.*
> *He was in the world and the world was made by*
> *Him, and the world knew Him not. . . .*
> *And the Word was made flesh, and dwelt amongst*
> *us.*

In the above statement of St. John, there cannot be any doubts about the nature of the Word. It is clearly the light and life of the world, the Creative Life-principle in which we live, move, and have our being. It is the Spirit of God, the very essence of the soul but now lost in the mighty swirl of the world and all that is worldly. It is only the contact with the Spirit that shows the way back to God and thus is the true religion. This contact is termed variously as the second birth, the resurrection, or the coming into life again. Addressing Nicodemus, a Pharisee and a ruler of the Jews, Jesus said:

> *Verily, verily, I say unto thee, except a man be born*

again, he cannot see the Kingdom of God....
(Mark the word "see.")
Verily, verily, I say unto thee, except a man be born
of water and of spirit, he cannot enter into the
Kingdom of God.... (Mark the word "enter.")
Marvel not that I said unto thee, ye must be born
again.

JOHN 3:3, 5, 7

Jesus compares the one born of the spirit with the wind which "bloweth where it listeth, for thou hearest the sound thereof, but canst not tell where it cometh, and whither it goeth" (John 3:8).

Elsewhere, he speaks of the holy Word as the "living water," the water that springs up into "everlasting life" (John 4:10, 14).

Jesus speaks of himself as the "bread of life," the "living bread" come down from heaven; and asks his disciples to eat "the flesh of the son of man, and drink his blood," for without these, "ye have no life in you" (John 6).

These in brief are the essential teachings of Christ, the Master Christian, but not of institutional Christianity. Most of the Christian doctrines were formulated not by Jesus but by St. Paul, who turned Christ into the sacrificial lamb to atone for the sins of the world, and around this central idea, as borrowed from Judaism and the cults flourishing around the Mediterranean at that time, there has grown a mass of ritual and ceremony.

The tenets of Christ remain as excellent moral precepts and doubtlessly point the way to the inner realization, but cannot in themselves put the seeker on the Path of realization, for they now lack the living impulse and the pulsating touch of the teacher, who having completed the job assigned to him in his own time, cannot now initiate and lead the people and make Truth real to them by bringing them face to face with Reality. Of all the mystical teachings of Christ, we now find but the symbolic lighting of candles in the churches and the ceremonial ringing of the big bell at the time of service. Few, if any, know the real significance behind these rituals, which are the outward representations of the twin principles of Light and Sound, or the primordial manifestations of the Godhead, responsible for all that exists in the Universe, seen and unseen. Some of the great church dignitaries, when asked, say that the bell is pulled simply to call men to prayer, and that to speak of God as the Father of Lights (James 1:17), is but a figurative form of speech to denote his greatest gifts (of the lights of reason and intellect). With hardly any experience of the inner truths, they take the words literally and try to explain things theoretically.

Jesus himself in no ambiguous words declared:

> I AM THE LIGHT OF THE WORLD: *he that followeth me shall not walk in darkness, but shall have the light of life.*
>
> JOHN 8:12

To speak of oneself as the "light of life" can have no reference to the light of the sun, even though the solar light may in the physical world be a source of life-giving energy. In Matthew 13:14, Jesus goes on to clarify the position and warns against literal interpretation of his words, when he draws the distinction between "hearing" and "understanding" and between "seeing" and "perception." It is only the awakened souls, the Masters of Truth, in living touch with the Reality, who hold the key to the Kingdom of the Spirit and can draw forth an individual, now completely lost in the life of the senses, and rediscover for him the great heritage of All-life and All-light, for then it is said that, "The eyes of the blind shall be opened and the ears of the deaf shall be unstopped. Then shall the lame man leap as an hart, and then the tongue of the dumb sing; for in the wilderness shall waters break out, and streams in the desert" (Isaiah 35:5-6).

How few of us really comprehend and appreciate the inner significance of the words of Jesus. We are content only with the ethical side of his teachings, which of course was a necessary accompaniment to the spiritual. The ethical tenets have been widely propagated and have even been assiduously kept alive, for they mark a great advance indeed in the moral scales of human values since the days of Moses. But by themselves, they fail to account for declarations like those about the "Day of Judgment," or "Repent, for the Kingdom of Heaven is at hand," or "God is Spirit and they that worship Him must worship Him in Spirit and in Truth." If such sayings were to be taken in their literal sense, it would be to reduce them to meaninglessness. The "Day of Judgment" has failed to come, in spite of the prophecy of its proximity, and either Christ was speaking in ignorance or we have failed to comprehend his real meaning. There is behind whatever he said always an inner meaning that is clear to those who have had the same mystic experiences, but baffle those who attempt to interpret it in terms of intellect or even intuition.

Not having direct inner perception (not to be confounded with philosophic speculation or intuitive insight), we attempt to interpret the significance of the teachings left to us in terms of our own limited experience. What was meant as a metaphor we take as literal, and the supersentient descriptions we reduce to metaphors. We easily forget that when Jesus said that he was "the light of the world," the "Son of God," and one who would not leave or forsake his disciples even unto the ends of the world, he spoke not in his mortal capacity, but like all other great Masters, as one who had merged with the Word and become one with It. Forgetting this, instead of following him on the spiritual path he showed, we think of him as a scapegoat for bearing our sins and as a means of evading the inner spiritual challenge.

III. Islam

As the name indicates, Islam is the religion of peace and good will for all who believe in the Prophet and follow his behests. Every religion that comes into being fulfills the purpose of God, the need of the hour, and fills a gap in the religious history of man. Prophet Mohammed too came at a time and in a place which was stinking with rank superstition, idolatry, social degradation and moral bankruptcy of the virile Arab race, debased as their brethren, the Jews, and other races had sometimes been. Both Arabs and Jews are Semitic in origin and are the descendants of Abraham: the one from Ishmael, banished eastward, and the other from his brother Isaac, who remained in the general area of Palestine. The rough and sturdy Bedouin tribes of the desert, owing allegiance to none but Mammon and Bacchus, were steeped in utter ignorance and given over heart and soul to warring against one another. It was to save such people that Mohammed, a deeply religious shepherd-boy, was chosen by the most High as His Elect, to carry out the fiat of the most Merciful among His creatures. The call to the Ministry of God came to him only after he had practiced intense spiritual discipline for several years in the rough and barren cave—Ghar-i-Hira— in the suburbs of Mecca.

He started his mission in the true spirit of humility, not to work wonders and offer miracles, which he always decried and desisted from, but as a simple preacher of God's words, a common man like anyone else. His message was essentially that of One God, for he emphatically declared:

There is no God but God and Allah is His Name.
Mohammed is but His messenger, or message-bearer.

On this fundamental basis of monotheism, he built his sys-

tem of ethical teachings and democratic brotherhood. This
was, indeed, the need of the time, and he admirably fulfilled
it. To the barbarous, crude and intellectually semi-developed
race, he could hardly offer metaphysical postulates for their
consideration, specially when even his simple teachings evoked
derision and ridicule from the people, and fierce vilification,
leading in time to open hostility, that forced him and his
followers to flee to Medina for safety. It was in the year
622 A.D. when the band of the faithful migrated from Mecca,
and was followed by a period of hard struggle for the newly
born faith, for the preservation and propagation of which, the
Prophet had to unsheath the sword in self-defense. The process of consolidation took about a hundred years of relentless
fighting, during which was carved a mighty empire from East
to West, the Indian Ocean on the one hand and the Atlantic
Ocean on the other.

The Koran or the Islamic Bible is a great wonder and an
outstanding miracle that surpassed everything else of that
period. It has one hundred and forty-four Suras or chapters,
each with verses varying from two hundred and eighty-six to
six, the number of verses going down in a descending order.
It is in an elegant and polished Arabic and was revealed in
parts to the unlettered Prophet when in moments of intense
meditation, by Gabriel the Archangel of God, whose voice,
originating in the reverberation of bells, would gradually assume sound, shape and form.

The simple teachings of the Koran center around *Allah*
(God), His *Makhluq* or the created world, *Insan* (Man)
and *Qiamat* or the doomsday. Since Allah is real and basically
good, so is everything else created by Him. As all life is individual, so everyone is to render an account for his deeds in
life, for he who wanders from the path has to bear the full
responsibility for his deviation in the after-life, on the day of
reckoning or *qiamat*.

The Path of peace and righteousness for Man is defined as one dedicated to (i) Allah or God; (ii) *Namaz* or prayer, which is enjoined at least five times a day whether standing, sitting, kneeling or lying down (to signify constant remembrance), and which may be performed anywhere by just spreading the prayer-carpet (*Sajadah*) and facing Mecca, the one common center of adoration for the faithful; (iii) *Zakaat* or charity of one-fourth of one's effect's once a year, for the poor and the needy, so that all may share jointly as members of the same human family; (iv) *Roza* or fast, during the month of Ramazan, so that the faithful may know what hunger is and learn to alleviate the sufferings of the hungry and also develop spiritual discipline, love of God, and compassion for their brethren, and lastly (v) *Haj* or performance of pilgrimage to Mecca, the Jerusalem of the faithful, at least once in one's lifetime, in simple sheet clothing, similar for all, thus making the rich and the poor alike, at least for the time being.

These in brief are the social teachings of Islam, designed for the betterment of the Arabic society. But there is in the Koran not much mention of the spiritual practices of the Prophet himself, which transformed a simple camel-driver into a Prophet-preacher and a statesman of high order. This once again brings into bold relief the ancient formula that there is some knowledge, by knowing which all else becomes known, that brings about complete identification with the heart of the Universe in a state of *maraqba* or meditation. We are told by the Master-saints that the practice in the solitary *Ghar-i-Hira* (cave of Hira), was no other than that of *Shughal-i-Nasiri,* or the Sound that works as an open sesame to the Kingdom of Allah.

Sheikh Mohd. Akram Sabri tells us that the Prophet practiced communion with *Awaz-i-mustqim* for fifteen years before he started receiving messages from God. We also learn that the Prophet accomplished *Shaqul-qamar,* i.e., he broke the moon in twain astride a milk-white charger *barq,* which figuratively and literally means lightning. These are clear indications of the inner spiritual experiences of those who travel the Path of the Sound Current and who know that they have to cross the star and the moon in their spiritual journey. Today, we see the symbolic representations of this in the star and the crescent moon on Muslim banners, Muslim coinage and postage stamps, etc. Again, the appearance of the moon on the *Id* days is always hailed with rejoicing and acclamation, and everywhere the people of the Mohammedan religion anxiously wait and watch from the housetops to see the dawning of the new moon on the horizon, little knowing the inner meaning that it conveys. Bound to the Book, they are rightly called the *Kitabis* or the people of the Book. Mohammed may be the last in the chain of the Prophets who have come, but the Koran enjoins one to seek some mediator for contact with God.

Apart from these references, we have the incontrovertible testimony of the Muslim mystics or *Sufis,* who have, in unmistakable words, spoken highly of the saving life-line as *Kalam-i-Qadim, Bang-i-Ilahi, Nida-i-Asmani, Saut-i-Sarmad,* all signifying the Abstract Sound (*Ism-i-Azam*), the one creative life-principle in all nature—the *Kalma,* which created fourteen *Tabaqs* or Regions. To this class of mystics belong Shamas Tabrez, Maulana Rumi, Hafiz Shirazi, Abdul Razaq Kashi, Inayat Khan, Baba Farid, Bulleh Shah, Shah Niaz, Hazrat Abdul Qadar, Hazrat Mian Mir, Hazrat Bahu, Hazrat Nizamud-din and many others, who all practiced *Sultan-ul-Azkar* (the highest Sound Principle). The *Fukra-i-Kamil,* travelers in the domain of *Marfat,* or true wisdom, bypass both *Shariat* and *Tariqat,* the paths of scripture, as well as *Hadis* or tradition.

Hazrat Inayat Khan in his book *The Mysticism of Sound*

speaks of the creation as the "Music of God," and tells us that *Saut-i-Sarmad* is the intoxicating vintage from the Garden of God.

All space, he says, is filled with Saut-i-Sarmad or the Abstract Sound. The vibrations of this Sound are too fine to be either audible or visible to the material ears or eyes, since it is even difficult for the eyes to see the form or color of the ether vibrations on the external plane. It was Saut-i-Sarmad, which Mohammed heard in the cave of Hira, when he became lost in his ideal. The Koran refers to it as *Kun-feu-kun*—Be and all became. Moses heard this very Sound on Koh-i-Toor or Mount Sinai, when in communion with God. The same Word was audible to Christ when absorbed in his heavenly Father in the wilderness. Siva heard the same *Anhad-Naad* in the Himalayas. The flute of Krishna is allegorically symbolic of the same Sound. This Sound is the source of all revelation to the Masters to whom it is revealed from within and, therefore, they know and teach the one and the same Truth for it is in this abstract reality that all the blessed ones of God unite.

This Sound of the Abstract is always going on within, around and about man. Those who are able to hear it and meditate on it are relieved from all worries, anxieties, sorrows, fears and diseases, and the soul is freed from the captivity of the senses and the physical body, and becomes part of the All-pervading Consciousness.

This Sound develops through and into ten different aspects, because of Its manifestation through the different tubes of the body (*Nadis*), and sounds like thunder, the roaring of the sea, the jingling of bells, the buzzing of bees, the twittering of sparrows, the vina, the flute, the sound of *Shankha* (conch) are heard, until It finally becomes *Hu,* the most sacred of all sounds, be they from man, bird, beast or thing.

In one of his addresses, Abdu'l-Baha said:

We must thank God that he has created for us both material blessings and spiritual bestowals. He has given us material gifts and spiritual graces; outer sight to view the light of the sun and inner vision by which we may perceive the Glory of God. He has designed the outer ear to enjoy the melodies of sound, and the inner hearing wherewith we may hear the Voice of our Creator.

In the *Hidden Words of Baha'u'llah*, a mystic saint of Persia, we have:

O Son of dust! hearken unto the mystic voice calling from the realm of the Invisible . . . up from thy prison, ascend unto the glorious meadows above and from thy mortal cage wing thy flight unto the paradise of the Placeless.

Many other Sufi mystics have sung likewise:

From the heavenly turret, God bids thee home,
Alas! thou listeneth not to the divine call,
None knows the mansion of the Beloved,
But sure enough the chiming of the bells comes from
*   there.*

KHWAJA HAFIZ

Rising above the horizon, hearken to the melody divine,
The prophet would attend to It as to any other task.

MAULANA RUMI

O God, lead me to the place from where flows the ineffable Kalma without words.

SHAH NIAZ

All repeat the Kalma by word of mouth,
A rare soul may do it with the tongue of thought,

He who communes with it mentally,
He can hardly describe it in words.

HAZRAT BAHU

In *Tazkra-i-Ghausia* (p. 332), Amir Khusro, a great mystic poet and a scholar of repute, has given an account of the ten types of sounds that one hears within, and he beautifully concludes with the following lines:

Such indeed is the Heavenly Orchestra, O Khusro,
It is in these ten melodies that a yogin gets absorbed.
With senses stilled and the mind at rest, so saith
  Khusro;
With the flourish of the limitless blast within,
All the lusts of the flesh and the deadly sins fly off,
The Master too has a wonderful world of His own,
And Khusro is now deeply engrossed within his self.

From the above, it is abundantly clear that the inner spiritual experience of the Sound Current is within the reach of an individual provided there is a competent Master who is capable of imparting his own life-impulse, and who can bring the consciousness in man to the center of his being and then into contact with the Light and Sound of God by opening the inner eye and by unsealing the inner ear.

Traces of these may now be found in the *Qawalis* or the outer music, and the raqs or dances with jingling anklets in which some of the Muslims engage to produce *Wajd*, a state of forgetfulness, as a means to the higher inner way.

IV. SIKHISM

Sikhism is the youngest of the world religions, tracing its origin from Guru Nanak, the first of the succession of ten great Gurus. Like other faiths, it assumed the character of a distinct religion only in subsequent times. Its Masters never claimed any novelty for their teachings. In fact, they laid great emphasis upon them as being the truths taught from time immemorial. To underline the universality of the spiritual message, Guru Arjan Dev (the fifth Guru), when compiling the *Sri Adi Granth,* the holy scripture of the Sikhs, drew the hymns and devotional pieces from the mystical writings of saints of all castes and creeds, including Kabir the Muslim weaver, Dhanna the *jat,* Ravi Das the cobbler and Sadna the butcher, etc.

The Sikh scriptures occupy a unique position in religious history. They represent not only the first deliberate attempt to present the oneness of all religions, but are composed in a language that is still alive and not a thing of the past. Hence they have lost none of their pristine freshness and have not been wholly buried under the debris of theological interpretation. Being mainly in the form of devotional lyrics, their appeal is not merely expositional. They speak of the whole man, singing of his problems, his weaknesses, the vanity of the world and the eternity of the Absolute, beckoning him on to greater and ever greater effort, toward his divine home. The language they employ lends itself to condensation—conjunctions being freely dispensed with—thus enabling its poetic and musical elements to be used with great effect. A searching philosophy and profound metaphysic are implicit in every statement, yet their writings speak directly to men's hearts in the language that they use, whose meanings are inexhaustible and which leave an imprint on all.

Moreover, the Sikh faith springing from the teachings not of one, but of a succession of great Masters, covers almost every major aspect of man's spiritual quest. If Buddha emphasized the need for moderation and non-attachment, Christ for love, the Sikh teachings succeed in stressing all facets. Besides, being of comparatively recent origin, the records of the personal lives of the ten great Gurus have been preserved, and we know much of their travels and actions. Nothing in a like manner is known of the Master-souls who gave to Hinduism its Upanishads. They speak as distant voices, reaching out to us from the remote past of mythology. The inner path is a practical one, and man needs not only philosophy but the demonstration of some life that illustrates it. Whether we read of the humility of Nanak as he passed on foot from place to place, bearing the spiritual torch, or of Gobind Singh, the last of the ten Gurus, riding from one end of the country to the other, organizing his followers into a brotherhood that could meet force with force and successfully resist the threat of physical extermination posed by the fanatical emperor Aurangzeb, we realize again and again that the life of God is inner perfection, a mode of being, a self-fulfillment, not to be confused with intellectual philosophy or metaphysical conundrums. He who had won this spiritual liberation could not be touched or tarnished by outer action, for he had made God's Will his own and did nothing of himself. And so, while leading his warriors to war against the Moguls, Guru Gobind Singh could yet sing:

> *Sach Kahun, sun leyo sabhay*
> *Jin prem kiyo, tin he Prabh payo.*
>
> *Verily, verily I say unto you*
> *They that loved, found the Lord.*

To attempt to outline the mystical message of the great Sikh Gurus would be to repeat most of what we have already said in the preceding chapter. For the teachings of Nanak and of Kabir (his contemporary), represent the final development of the mysticism of inner seeing and hearing into the Path of the Surat Shabd Yoga. Both great Masters—one the first of the line of Sikh Gurus and the second a weaver of Varanasi (formerly Benares), were indefatigable in emphasizing the inefficacy of outer ritual, intellectual sophistication and yogic austerities:

Sant mata kuchh aur hai Chhado chaturai

The path of the Masters is distinct;
Let go thy intellectual subtleties.

KABIR

One cannot comprehend Him through reason, even
*   if one reasoned for ages;*
One cannot achieve inner peace by outward silence,
*   not though one sat dumb for ages;*
One cannot buy contentment with all the riches of
*   the world, nor reach Him with all mental inge-*
*   nuity.*

NANAK

Both saints decried caste distinctions, and they were alike in stressing the unity of all life, the oneness of the spirit that sustained everything, and both declared repeatedly that the highest and most feasible way to at-one-ment with God lay through the path of *Naam* or *Shabd*. Indeed, no other scriptures are so insistent on the all-pervasiveness of the Word as are those of the Sikhs or the writings of Kabir, a selection of which, as has already been mentioned, was included by Guru Arjan Dev in the Sri Adi Granth. The inner light—*antar jot* —and the inner music—*panch shabd,* or the five-melodied Word, whose music is limitless (*anhad bani*), are a recurring theme in nearly all of the compositions contained in the Granth Sahib.

The Jap Ji by Guru Nanak, which figures as a prologue to the Granth Sahib, may serve to illustrate the spiritual riches embedded in the Sikh scriptures. It is a wonderful lyrical composition, remarkable for its poetic beauty, and even more for the divine heights it reaches. It opens by dwelling on the nature of the Absolute Reality as distinct from the phenomenal:

> *There is one Reality, the Unmanifest Manifested;*
> *Ever-existent, He is Naam (Conscious Spirit);*
> *The Creator pervading all;*
> *Without fear, without enmity;*
> *The Timeless, the Unborn and the Self-existent,*
> *Complete within Itself.*
>
> PROLOGUE

This Reality is beyond human reason and comprehension:

> *One cannot comprehend Him through reason, even*
> *if one reasoned for ages.*
>
> STANZA I

And yet, It may be reached, and the path leading to It is single:

> *There is a Way, O Nanak: to make His Will our*
> *own,*
> *His Will which is already wrought in our existence.*
>
> STANZA I

It is not something outside of us, but within; it is a part of our being, our very essence, and all that is needed is to attune ourselves to It, for to be attuned to It is to be freed from the bondage of the ego and therefore of maya:

> *All exist under His Will,*
> *And nothing stands outside,*
> *One attuned with His Will, O Nanak, is wholly freed*
> *from ego.*
>
> STANZA II

How may one attune oneself to the divine Will? The answer is hinted at in the very opening itself:

> *Through the favor of His true servant the Guru,*
> *He may be realized.*

This subject is taken up in Stanza XVI in greater detail:

> *The saint (the Word-personified) is acceptable at*
> *His Court and is the chief elect therein;*
> *The saint adorns the threshold of God and is honored*
> *even by kings;*
> *The saint lives by and meditates on the One Word.*

The gift of the true Master is a gift of *Naam*, in which he himself is an adept. This Word is the manifestation of God's Will and Command and is at the heart of all His creations:

> *With one Word of His, this vast creation blossomed*
> *into being,*
> *And a thousand streams of life sprang into existence.*
>
> STANZA XVI

The way to at-one-ment with God's Will is through attunement with the Word:

> *By communion with the Word one becomes the*
> *abode of all virtues;*
> *By communion with the Word, one becomes a*
> *Sheikh, a Pir and a true spiritual king;*
> *By communion with the Word, the spiritually blind*
> *find their way to Realization;*
> *By communion with the Word, one crosses beyond*
> *the Limitless Ocean of illusionary matter;*
> *O Nanak! His devotees live in perpetual ecstasy,*
> *for the Word washes away all sin and sorrow.*
>
> STANZA XI

Hence it is that Nanak declares:

Exalted is the Lord, and exalted His abode;
More exalted still His Holy Word.

STANZA XXIV

Having outlined the nature of the Absolute and the way
leading to mergence with It, Nanak goes on to tell us of what
is required to successfully pursue the journey. It is not necessary, he implies, to turn an outward sanyasin; what one must
do is to be a sanyasin in spirit, dispensing with external forms,
and instead to inculcate the inner virtues:

Let contentment be your ear-rings;
Endeavor for the Divine and respect for the Higher
  Self be your wallet;
And constant meditation on Him your ashes;
Let preparedness for death be your cloak,
And your body be like unto a chaste virgin;
Let your Master's teachings be your supporting staff.
The highest Religion is to rise to Universal Brother-
  hood,
  Aye, to consider all creatures your equals.
Conquer your mind, for victory over self is victory
  over the world.
Hail, Hail, to Him alone,
The Primal, Pure, Eternal, Immortal and Immu-
  table in all ages.

STANZA XXVIII

Finally, in the closing sections of the Jap Ji, Guru Nanak
gives us a bird's-eye view of the spirit's pilgrimage. The first
realm to be transcended is the plane of *Dharm Khand*—the
Realm of Action, or the world of good and evil deeds as we

know it. Next comes *Gyan Khand* or the Realm of Knowledge, the first of the inner heavens, full of gods and demi-gods:

> *Countless its elements, air, water and fire,*
> *And countless Krishnas and Sivas,*
> *And countless the Brahmas fashioning various crea-*
> *tions of countless forms and countless hues.*
> *Countless the Fields of Action, countless the golden*
> *mountains . . .*
> *Countless the sources of creation, countless the har-*
> *monies, countless those that listen unto them.*
> *And countless the devotees of the Word,*
> *Endless and unending, O Nanak! this Realm.*
>
> STANZA XXXV

If knowledge is the reigning virtue of this region, ecstasy is that of the next, which is *Sarm Khand,* the Realm of Bliss. This plane is beyond description and whoever tries to describe it must repent his folly. Herein at last, the soul is freed from its mental adjuncts and finally comes into its own:

> *Herein the mind, reason and understanding are ethe-*
> *realized, the self comes to its own, and develops the*
> *penetration of the gods and the sages.*
>
> STANZA XXXVI

But "higher still" stands *Karm Khand,* the Realm of Grace—grace earned through right action and meditation.

> *Here the Word is all in all, and nothing else prevails,*
> *Here dwell the bravest of the brave, the conquerors*
> *of the mind, imbued with the love Divine . . .*
> *All hearts filled with God, they live beyond the reach*
> *of death and of delusion.*
>
> STANZA XXXVII

This is the realm where the soul finally escapes the coils of relativity; the bonds of time, death and change, no longer affect it. But though it dwells in the constant presence of the Lord, it may move still further to merge into His Formless State:

> *Sach Khand, or the Realm of Truth, is the seat of*
> *the Formless One,*
> *Here He creates all creations, rejoicing in creating.*
> *Here are many regions, heavenly systems and uni-*
> *verses,*
> *To count which were to count the countless.*
> *Here, out of the Formless,*
> *The heavenly plateaux and all else come into form,*
> *All destined to move according to His Will.*
> *He who is blessed with this vision, rejoices in its*
> *contemplation.*
> *But, O Nanak, such is its beauty that to try to*
> *describe it is to attempt the impossible.*
>
> STANZA XXXVII

The world shall go on along the rails of good and evil deeds, caught in the limits of Karma, but:

> *Those who have communed with the Word, their*
> *toils shall end,*
> *And their faces shall flame with glory.*
> *Not only shall they have salvation,*
> *O Nanak, but many more shall find freedom with*
> *them.*
>
> FINALE

Such was the lofty message not only of Guru Nanak, but also of his successors. Their word blazed like a summer fire through the plains of the Punjab, sweeping away all the false distinctions of caste that a decadent Brahminism had created. At a time when religious bigotry between the Hindus and the ruling Muslims was growing, it demonstrated the unity of all true religions, purifying Hinduism of its servility to outer ritual and setting up before Islam the higher inner ideal it was forgetting in outer names and forms. It is no accident that the Sufi tradition and the Sikh religious movement should have flowered at the same time. Indeed, history at many points, suggests an active cooperation between the two. Some of the Sikh Gurus, especially Guru Nanak and Guru Gobind Singh, and their followers like Bhai Nand Lal, were masters of Persian and have left some exquisite compositions in that language. Guru Nanak is said to have journeyed to Mecca and, like his successors, had many Muslim disciples, while Sufi mystics like Hazrat Mian Mir were on intimate terms with Guru Arjan. Both the Sufi and the Sikh Masters were not tied to dogma, and taught the lesson of universal brotherhood. They acted and reacted upon each other, and it is significant that the Surat Shabd Yoga, or the Yoga of the Sound Current, should find equal stress in the writings of the greatest Sufis and in the Sikh scriptures, a fact summed up by Inayat Khan in the passage already quoted from his book *The Mysticism of Sound.*

But the teachings of all great Masters tend to trail off into institutions after they leave this world. Those of the Sikh Gurus have been no exception to the rule. While they still exercise a profoundly uplifting influence upon the masses, they no longer impel them to mystic efforts as they once must have done. That which once sought to transcend all religious divisions has itself become a religion. That which sought to castigate caste and caste-emphasis has gradually developed a certain caste-consciousness. That which sought to break through all outer forms and ritual has cultivated a form and ritual of its own. At every religious ceremony, people hear verses chanted, singing of the glories within:

> *All knowledge and meditation sprang from Dhun*
> *(the Sound Principle),*
> *But what That is, defies definition.*
>
> GURU NANAK

> *The true Bani (Word) is given by the Guru,*
> *And is reverberating in the Sukhmana.*
>
> GURU ARJAN

> *The Unstruck Music is heard through the Grace of*
> *a Godman,*
> *But few there be who commune with it.*
>
> GURU NANAK

> *Perfect is the Anhad Bani (Limitless Song),*
> *And Its key is with the Saints.*
>
> GURU ARJAN

And yet these verses are chanted without heeding or understanding the deep spiritual meaning hidden in them.

CHAPTER SEVEN

Some Modern Movements

THE first impact of science on the West seems to have been to undermine religion. Christianity, having developed into a complex and rigid institution with a dogmatic framework, was in no position to adjust itself to the demands made by the new knowledge available from science. The result was unavoidable; a head-on collision between the two, which left religion shaken, and science firmly entrenched. However, as we have already suggested in an earlier chapter, the physical sciences by themselves cannot explain life completely or even adequately. When the outer sciences have had their say, certain unknown problems of being remain to baffle and trouble the mind of man. The last century has seen the emergence of many a movement that has sought, in some way or other, to point toward an inner life, that science at least to a degree tended to discount. Modern India has been the birthplace of many religious movements, but for the most part they have been by way of a revival of what the ancients already knew, be it the Vedantism of Sri Ramakrishna, Sri Aurobindo, or Ramana Maharshi or, as we have already examined in some detail, the various Indian yogic systems. However, it may be fruitful to glance at some of the movements prevalent in the West, movements that often converge on Eastern traditions and are affected by them.

Roscrucianism, Theosophy and "I Am" Activity

Even while Christianity held unquestioned sway in Europe, certain heterodox schools of mysticism flourished in a small way alongside it, Rosicrucianism being one of the earliest. However, these continued as secret societies which were looked upon with suspicion by the general public. But when institutional Christianity began to suffer at the hands of science, they suddenly acquired an importance that they never had before. Men whose faith in Christianity had been shaken by Darwin and Huxley but who could not accept the mechanistic view of the Universe, turned to these societies in the hope of arriving at a more satisfying explanation of life. Many took to the tenets of Rosicrucianism while others, seeking their inspiration from the East, founded the Theosophical movement. Still others, claiming to be guided by St. Germain, have developed what is called the "I Am" Activity. These movements do not claim to be religions in the traditional sense, even though they have their own codes. They are rather occult societies which share in common a belief that human life is guided and directed by unseen Cosmic Beings or Mystical Brotherhoods. These Beings cannot be met directly in this physical world; they either live in remote mountain fastnesses or work from a plane higher than the earthly one. However, one may, by believing in them and by following a particular discipline, lend oneself to their influence and benefit thereby. Though they all imply, in one way or another, the ultimate unity of life, in practice they seem to touch it at its fringes. The most a disciple may hope to do is to get in direct touch with one of the Cosmic Beings, but that state in which the soul becomes one with the Source of Time and the Timeless, of which the great Masters have spoken, is seldom treated as a practical possibility. Again, since one seeks guidance not from a human being like oneself, who has realized the Infinite, but from visionary beings whom one may never meet, the kind of detailed instruction and step by step guidance in every field of life, which is an essential feature of the Surat Shabd Yoga, is also missing. However, each in its own way seeks to carry human evolution a step further, and the step taken is certainly not a mean one. Thus, Madam Blavatsky, writing in *The Voice of the Silence,* speaks of a fairly advanced mystic experience when describing the inner Sound:

> *The first is the nightingale's sweet voice chanting a song of parting to its mate. The second comes as a sound of silver cymbals of the Dhyanis awakening the twinkling star. The next is plaint-melodies of the ocean spirit imprisoned in its shell. And this is followed by the chant of Vina. The fifth, like the sound of a bamboo flute shrills in the ears. It changes into a triumphant blast. The last vibrates like the dull rumbling of thunder clouds.*

Christian Science and Subud

The Christian Science movement is yet another heterodox Western movement, but it differs from those that we have already noticed in its shift of emphasis. Though it implies a mystical base, yet in practice it is not very much concerned with it. It seeks to interpret Christ's life in its own light, focusing its attention simply on the miracles performed by him. It argues that God, or the Truth, is good, and that all evil and disease are but a result of losing contact with this Inner Power. He who can be put in touch with it can be cured of all disease, and Christian Science has tended to concentrate its attention on this end. The result has been that it has become more a study of health than one of spiritual evolution, and the line between healing through auto-suggestion and hypnotic suggestion, and healing (as Christian Science claims) through the power of Truth is not always easy to draw. Many have even questioned the nature of the motives of its founder, Mrs. Mary Baker Eddy. But of one thing one can be certain: that even if the cures effected by Christian Science spring from a spiritual source, the agents are not its conscious masters, are not in direct and conscious contact with the higher power, but act as its unconscious instruments.

Though it would be rash to class with Christian Science *Subud* or *Soshiel Bodhi Dharm,* founded by the Indonesian mystic teacher Pak Subeh, which has now become an international movement, yet one may with some justice notice a similar trend. The mystic base in the case of Subud is much more important than in that of Christian Science, yet is often directed toward the same end. It seeks, through following a certain course of exercises called *Latihan,* to put its followers in touch with hidden psychic powers. It does not seem to enhance consciousness directly but enriches it indirectly through increasing one's powers of intuition. Whether one looks at the experiences of Mohammad Raufe or those of John Bennett, one realizes that in the case of Subud, a person may serve as a medium for higher spiritual forces, curing people of diseases, without becoming a conscious co-worker. The result is that instead of progressing to higher and still higher planes of consciousness, until one merges with the Infinite, one tends to cultivate a passive receptivity to psychic powers which may not necessarily be of the higher kind. Many disciples during Latihan reproduce strange animal or bird experiences—a far cry from the Nirvikalp Samadhi or the Sehaj Samadhi spoken of by the greatest mystics.

Spiritism and spiritualism

Last but not the least, we must distinguish spirituality from spiritism and spiritualism, as spirituality is quite different from both of them. Spiritism inculcates a belief in the existence of disembodied spirits apart from matter, which are believed by those who believe in spiritism to haunt either the nether regions as ghosts or evil spirits, or even as angels or good spirits in the lower astral regions. At times, they even become interested in the individual human affairs, and for the fulfillment of long-cherished but unfulfilled desires, try to seek gratification by all sorts of tricks, and those who dabble in the Black Art claim and profess to exercise power over them through magical incantations. But none of the Master's disciples need bother about them, as no evil influence can come near one who is in communion with the holy Word, for it is said:

> *The Great Angel of Death is an invincible foe,*
> *But he too fears to come near one in communion*
> *with the Word.*
> *He flies far out and away from the chants of the*
> *divine Harmony,*
> *Lest he fall a victim to the wrath of the Lord.*

Spiritualism goes one step further than spiritism. It is a belief in the survival of the human personality after physical death, and the possibility of communication between the living and the dead. The advocates of spiritualism very often hold seances for getting into communication with so-called spirits. Their modus operandi is by mediumship, for they work through some sort of medium, maybe a planchette for planchette writing, a table for table rapping, or even a human being who is rendered unconscious so that the spirit called may make use of his body and communicate through it. This relationship generally works between just the physical or earth plane and the lowest sub-astral planes known as magnetic fields. The results that follow from such communications are very limited in scope, mostly unreliable and extremely harmful to the medium, who suffers a terrible loss at times by deprivation of his intelligence. The Masters of spirituality, therefore, strongly condemn the practice of spiritualism. Their contact and intercourse with the spiritual regions right to the mansion of the Lord (Sach Khand) are direct and they come and go at their sweet will and pleasure, without any let or hindrance and independent of the subjective process of mediumship.

While their approach is quite normal, natural, direct and constructive, the spiritualist on the other hand works subjectively, indirectly, and mediately through a process which is fraught with dangers and risks both to himself and to the medium. Spiritualism, apart from the knowledge of survival of spirits after death, adds little to our experience and offers nothing of substance in the way of spirituality.

Hypnosis and mesmerism

The above remarks apply equally to hypnosis and mesmerism, in both of which a person with a stronger will power tries to influence those with weaker stamina by means of passes of hand or gestures coupled with a riveted attention on the subject. In certain ailments, like hysteria, etc., some physicians also make use of these processes and are able temporarily to effect cures and alleviate pains and aches for which they are not able to find a proper remedy.

Spirituality, on the contrary, is the science of the soul, and consequently, it deals with all the aspects of the soul, where it resides in the human body, its relationship with the body and with the mind, how it seemingly acts and reacts through and on the senses, its real nature, and how it can be separated from all its finitizing adjuncts. It describes the spiritual journey with its wealth of spiritual planes and sub-planes, the spiritual powers and possibilities and their intrinsic worth. Spirituality discloses what the holy Word is and how to commune with It, tells us that the ultimate goal is Self-realization and God-realization, or the union of the soul with the Over-soul, and teaches how it can be achieved by means of Surat Shabd Yoga or the Path of the Sound Current, as described in the foregoing pages.

CHAPTER EIGHT

Conclusion

THE foregoing survey, in brief, of the major religions of the world and some of their modern ramifications, makes abundantly clear a general drift toward some common basic assumptions and beliefs: (a) that the physical universe is no more than a small part of a much larger whole; (b) that in like manner, our everyday human existence is only a fragment of the vast and complex pattern of life; (c) that behind the phenomenal, physical and human world, there is an Absolute Reality or a state of Perfect Being, beyond change or destruction, complete within Itself, which is responsible for all that is and yet stands over and above Its own creation; (d) that this Reality, this state of Perfect Being, may be approached by man (under competent guidance) through the agency of the Word, or the Divine stream radiating Light and Harmony, which represent the primal manifestations of the Formless into Form and from whose downward descent all realms and regions came into existence.

If all religious experience tends in the same direction, then why, one asks, is there so much of conflict and controversy in the sphere of religion? Why is it that the devotees of every faith regard theirs as the only true one and all other faiths as false? Why is there dogmatic faith in spiritual monopoly and wherefore the Holy Crusades, the Massacre of St. Bartholomew, the Spanish Inquisition or the communal riotings in India in 1947? The question is a valid one, and the reasons that must go toward answering it are many and complex.

The first thing that strikes one when taking up the compara-

236

tive study of religion is its existence on different levels. At the core of every major religion stands the practical, mystical experience of some great sage or a succession of sages. Around this center have accumulated accretions of social codes, customs and ritual. Now the core may be common to the mystics of various ages and countries, but the social context in which it is experienced and conveyed must of necessity vary. The Westerner bares his head as a mark of reverence, while the Oriental covers it. The Hindu, belonging to a land with many rivers and abundant water, bathes before his prayers, while his Muslim counterpart, coming from the deserts of Arabia, is satisfied with a dry bath with sand. The European, living as he does in the colder regions, feels neither of these compulsions. Such differences of custom extend to other spheres as well. Polygamy may be lawful to the Muslim but it is a sin to the Catholic. Idol worship may be quite permissible in Hinduism but is hateful to the Puritan. The fact is that all religious leaders have stressed the need for maintaining high ethical standards, but their ethic has never been of the nature of an absolute. They have taken into account the social conditions obtaining among the people at the times at which they came and have tried to raise them to the highest possible point, aiming not so much at a standardization of outer custom as at inner purity of heart, and good will toward one's human and non-human fellow creatures. Jesus' immediate listeners may have failed to appreciate the truth of his assertion that he had come not to "break" but to "fulfill" the Law, and yet if Moses gave out the precept of "an eye for an eye and a tooth for a tooth," Christ taught his disciples to love their enemies and to offer their right cheek when the left was slapped. Moses spoke according to the conditions of his time, and Jesus according to his own, so the ethics of Christianity deviated from those of Judaism, even though it is an extension of the older faith.

As a consequence of the factors that came into play in the development of religion as a social institution, we find that each religion creates around itself a distinct pattern of customs, dogmas and ritual. This pattern being distinct in each case, the devotees of every faith must necessarily feel themselves as standing apart from those of other faiths, not only in their dress and manners, but also in their modes of social concepts and attitudes. Yet the lives of all great religious leaders like Jesus and Buddha, reveal that while each of them accepted and extended the code of his own people, they nonetheless never forgot that all men were brothers and treated members of other societies with the same respect and consideration as they displayed to those of their own. Behind the varying outer forms that characterize life they saw pulsating the same Unity of Being, and it was from this level that they regarded all humanity.

What was possible to the great founders of religions should be possible for those who claim to follow them. But when we look at things as they stand, we find that this possibility of inter-communication, cooperation and understanding between various faiths, has seldom if ever been realized. A mystic like Sri Ramakrishna may practically demonstrate the inner oneness of all religions,* but the rest of us fail to grasp the point. The fact is that every major world religion, after the passing away of its founder, grew into an institution, with a priesthood to manage its affairs: the pundits in India, the *Mullahs* and *Maulvis* in Islam, the pharisees and rabbis in Judaism and the monks and bishops in Christianity. This development made possible the extension of the message of the great founders to numbers they could never have instructed themselves. Buddha personally met and influenced many an indi-

---

* Sri Ramakrishna, to test the truth that all religions lead to the same spiritual goal, practiced in turn the outer and inner disciplines of Hinduism, Christianity and Islam, and in each case, he found the end reached was the same.

vidual, but what was their number in comparison to the millions that heard the doctrine of Dharma when Ashoka created the various *Sanghas* or orders of Buddhist monks, two centuries after his death? Besides, it enabled the perpetuation of his message down the ages. Buddha has come and gone, Jesus may have been immolated on the cross, but the Sangh and the Church continue and keep alive their teachings in a widespread manner, which could not have been done if no such institutions had been developed.

But, if the institutionalization of the teachings of great spiritual leaders enabled their propagation and perpetuation, it also led to their transformation. The message of Christ or of Buddha as it was first delivered by each of them was one thing, but in the hands of the Church and Sangh that followed, it became another. The great religious leaders were moved and guided by first-hand inner experience and it was this actuality that lay at the heart of their teachings. They saw it as something universal, something latent in every man, and it was toward this that they directed the attention of their disciples, employing ethical advancement as a lever for spiritual progress. When their task, after their passing away, was taken over by rapidly expanding organizations, which grew more complex with time, one could not expect all of their members to have attained the same heights or even to have any glimpses of the inner mystic realms. Little wonder then, that with the growth of the church and the like, the interest in every religion should have tended to shift from the mystical to the ethical, the ritualistic and the doctrinal; in short, from the universal to the particular. Only a rare soul may penetrate through the dark veil within, but for every such being, a million, nay a billion, may discuss problems of ethics, practice outer ceremonies and hold strong opinions on various subjects, opinions not inspired or tested by personal experience, but picked up from the marketplace of life. And so, whereas we find no rigid framework of ritual or doctrine or outer code in the teachings of Jesus himself—everything being fluid and flexible, in a ready state to be directed to the service of the mystical message—a rigid framework emerged with the growth of the Christian Church. As this variation took place, new barriers arose between the followers of Jesus and those of other faiths, barriers that never existed before.

As though this were not enough, the rise of priestcraft worked in yet another direction. The Church in its phase of growth had, in most cases, to struggle against heavy odds, as everything new usually meets with strong opposition. It could only offer the cross of danger and deprivation, not the rose of prosperity. Those who entered it, entered it for the sake of their convictions, not for love of power. But once the Church had come to be accepted, it began to exercise considerable sway over the people. They offered it gifts and titles and made it the final arbiter, not only in matters spiritual, but in matters temporal as well. Thus began a process by which the priesthood turned from the inner to the outer life, from self-abnegation to temporal power. In order to preserve its position, the Church encouraged the growth of doctrines and traditions, that reinforced its monopoly of authority. To strengthen itself, it created a halo around the altar to which it was in service, and condemned the altars where it had no hand. If the self-styled servants of Jehovah, or those of some other name of deity, were to maintain and extend their position and sway, then it was necessary that all gods of the philistines or of the heathens should be condemned.

These factors that we have considered operate in every field of human activity. The historian is only too well aware of the fate of every new movement, whether of a religious or of a secular character. It arises with a man of vision, undergoes rapid expansion in the hands of those whom his example has directly inspired, and then enters into a process of gradual senility and decay. The descent from a pulsating vision to a mechanical dogma is not peculiar to religion alone, but nevertheless there are certain features in the case of religion which do not occur elsewhere.

These unique problems stem from the mystical experience at the heart of every great religion. The mystic experience, as we have seen, extends to planes of existence to which normally human beings have no access. Only a handful, nay less than a handful, can claim its mastery in any age. It is an experience unique in character, for it possesses a kind of richness, extensiveness, intensity and beauty that finds no parallel in earthly life. But we on this earthly plane can comprehend its meaning only within the limitations of our own mundane experience. The choice before the mystic, if he wishes to convey to us something of his unique experience (not just ending in silence or in the negative statements of the Vedantist or of St. John of the Cross), is perforce to resort to metaphor and parable.

In Maulana Rumi's Masnavi, we are told:

It is not fitting that I tell thee more,
For the stream's bed cannot hold the sea.

Jesus was quite explicit on the subject when speaking to his closest disciples (to whom he could directly convey firsthand inner experience):

Unto you it is given to know the mystery of the
Kingdom of God; but unto those that are without,
all things are done in parables.

ST. MARK

Whereas direct statement tends to be limited by the analyzable qualities of the object, figurative statement suffers no such bar. Poets have described their love for a woman in terms of a rose, a star, a melody, a flame, the moon, etc. The mystics have used a similar license when speaking of their love for God. But while the listeners to the poet speaking of human love are always aware that he is using metaphors, knowing well what a woman is, those hearing the mystic have no such comparison and often tend to forget that what he is saying is only figurative. So the statements of the man of spiritual vision are often taken literally when they are meant to be only metaphorical, and metaphorically when they are meant to be literal. Thus, when Jesus or Mohammed declared that he was the son or the messiah of God (as all great souls who have merged their will with the Divine Will have said), they were each taken to imply that he was literally the only son of the Almighty. Or again, when Jesus, speaking not in his capacity as a finite individual but in that of the Eternal Divine Principle that he embodied, said, "I shall never leave thee nor forsake thee even to the ends of the world," he was taken literally. So to seek active spiritual guidance from a living teacher after Jesus was no more, became a sign of disbelief and therefore was dubbed a heresy. But when Jesus quite literally spoke of the "single eye" or of God as "Light," he was taken to refer figuratively to integrity of conscience and the light of reason.

Little wonder then that with each statement being thus interpreted, or rather misinterpreted, meanings should emerge which the sage who made them never had in mind, and dogmas and doctrines should be propounded in his name which have little relation to the universal inner experiences which inspired him. So differences of doctrine between one creed and another arose that were never in the contemplation of their founders. Moreover, the inner realms are so vast and varied that no one mystic could ever hope to point to all aspects of the inner panorama. At best he can hint at some part of it and that may not be exactly the same as those parts of which others have spoken, with the result that to the reader who has himself no direct access to the realms within, there may appear certain discrepancies between the writings of one mystic and another, which in fact do not exist.

Further, not all mystics reach the highest spiritual goal. Only a few succeed in breaking through the veil of inner darkness to the full, and of these, the majority never get beyond the first inner spiritual plane. Of those who do succeed in going further, the greater number never cross the second plane, and so on. Now each of the planes has its own peculiarities and characteristics and, whereas the higher planes contain and maintain the lower ones, the inhabitants of the lower planes are seldom aware of the existence of the higher ones. Each plane, in comparison to the one before it, seems perfection itself, and every mystic who has spoken of his divine experience, has described it as though it were the be-all and the end-all of spiritual progress. The inescapable consequence of this is that we encounter descriptions of the Absolute that, after an allowance for differences of figurative language has been made, fail to agree. Jesus speaks of the Divine in Its paternal aspect, Sri Ramakrishna in Its maternal one. The Sankhya mystics speak of God, Prakriti and Atman as forever separate; Ramanuja as related but never merging into one; while Shankara sees them as of the selfsame essence, their separation being not real but only an illusion. All this means a mass of confusion to the common reader. But should he meet one who has reached the highest realm and is familiar with the experience of each of the inner planes, all contradictions would vanish, for he can demonstrate that though the six blind men made apparently the most contradictory statements about the nature of the elephant, yet they could all be finally reconciled by one who could see the whole elephant.

In this context, the teachings of the Surat Shabd Yoga acquire yet another significance. We have already seen at some length how it represents the quickest, most practical and the most scientific means to man's spiritual goal. We may now add that by taking him to the highest of the spiritual planes, the point where the Formless comes into Form, it provides him with the best vantage-ground for viewing the vast field of spirituality. That which would confuse and baffle others leaves the adept on this Path unruffled. Contradictions vanish at his touch, and that which once confused and confounded resolves itself, after his exposition, into perfect order. He understands each of the spiritual and quasi-spiritual movements that confront us today. He can at will enter into the inner experience that each can offer, and he is the best fitted to judge their relative merits. He does not condemn or attack; he is not moved by hatred or opposition. Having seen the Highest, his aim is to take his fellow human beings to It in the smoothest, swiftest way. He knows that the life within is not to be confounded with the life without, and preaches his message not as a code but as a science: "Try within," he tells us, "and see for yourself."

The science he teaches is not a new one. It is the most ancient of sciences. But whereas in the past it tended to ally itself to much that was not essential to it, he wishes to preserve it in its pure state and pristine glory. He carries to their logical conclusion the mystic truths embedded in all great scriptures, stressing that if God in His primal form is Light and Music, we must inwardly turn to these, and not to any other means, for reaching back to Him and merging with Him. Where there was chaos he brings order, where there was despair he brings hope, and for each of us, in whatever capacity we may be, he has some comfort, some illumination to offer.

INDEX

Index

The foreign terms listed below are mostly defined in the text, usually when first mentioned. The asterisk (*) marks definitions or explanations in depth.

246

250 THE CROWN OF LIFE

Jehovah, 240
Jerusalem, 215
Jesus, 151, 169, 170, 241-143
Jews, 213
Jewish, 29
Jiva, conditioned soul, 22;* embodied soul, 23;* contacted with past Masters, 69; separated from conditioned state, 81; seems separated from Bhahman, 114; realizes one-ness, 122; same essence as atman, 125,* 130;* helped by a Satguru, 160,* 173, 179*
Jiva-atma, 77
Jivan-mukta, 17, 131, 159
Jnana (also, Gyan), a veil over soul, 78;* concealing a higher state, 79;* gives no freedom beyond itself, 138; within ability of few, 139; subordinate to the power of Shabd, 142
Jnana chakshu, 77
Jnana Yoga, 5, 6, 18, 103, 104-106,* 139
Jnani, 79, 112, 139
Jonson, Ben, 5, 76
Judaism, 210, 237-238
Jyoti, 114, 143

Kabir, 66, 71, 74, 85, 125, 162, 166, 167, 220, 221
Kabir Panthies, 68
Kaivalya, 38
Kaivalya Samadhi, 77
Kala & Mahakala, 139, 142
Kal, 114
Kalam-i-Qadim, 216
Kali, 161
Kalma, 101, 129, 145, 187,* 216, 218
Kanth chakra, 65, 63, 68, 71, 78
Karm Khand, 226
Karma, freed from binding effects, 7; knowledge of, 57; kinds of, 75; importance of freedom from, 104; as a form of yoga, 109-111; action by a bound jiva

creates even more, 130; realm beyond, 227
Karm Kshetra, 7, 104
Karma Yoga, 5, 7, 109-111*
Karma Yogin, 111, 112, 137
Karmic vibrations, 179
Katha Upanishad, 60, 101
Khat Shastras, 20
Khechari Muda, 36, 37,* 56, 77
Khusro, 168, 219
knower, 124, 126
knowing, 132*
knowing mind, 126*
knowledge, 13, 103, 104, 115, 120,* 123, 125-131; of mind, 55; realm of, 226
Koh-i-toor, 155, 217
Koran, 214-217
Koshas, 13,* 14, 16, 17, 47, 71-73, 78-81, 99, 100, 158
Krishna, 100, 102-104, 112, 195, 211,* 222
Kriyas, 67, 91
Kshar, 93n.
Kumbhaka, 46, 47, 67
Kundalini, 47, 99
Kundalini Shakti, 67
Kundalinic energy, 164

Lao Tze, 199
Latihan, 233
Lavanya, 59
Laya Yoga, 86, 97-99,* 137
liberated soul, 17
liberation, 75, 100, 110, 119, 179
liberation, spiritual, 221
life, 68
life current, 10,* 11
life of God, 221
life stream, 187*
light, 70,* 73,* 120, 123, 129, 142-145, 147, 155, 159, 160, 178, 181, 189, 195, 205, 206, 209, 211*
lion, 174-175
Lion roar of Dharma, 197-198
lobh, 48, 149
Logos, 129,* 143,* 189
lotus, 54, 64, 66

Vedantism, 48, 230
Vedantists, 88
Vedas, 88, 102, 128
Vedic Age, 88, 190
Vedic Hymns, 191
Vedic Mantras, 88,* 193, 194
Vedic Pantheon, 197
vegetarian, 151, 152
vibrations, 77, 88, 102, 179, 198, 217*
Videha, 56, 74
Videh Mukti, 115, 159
Vidya, 124
Vigyan, 13, 18, 165
Vigyanic energy, 154
Vigyanic system, 165
Vigyan mai, 61, 68, 71, 73, 78, 79, 80
Vigyan mai jivas, 80
Vigyan mai kosh, 13, 71
Vishnu, 102, 161, 171
Vishuddhi Chakra, 55
Vishvamitra, 59
Vivek, 112
Vivekananda, Swami, 30, 121
Viyog, 20
Void, 36, 38
Vritis, 4, 6, 7,* 8,* 33,* 48, 50, 126, 127*
Vyasa, 101

waking, 123, 124, 193
water of life, 210
We Wei, 202
wisdom, 125, 216
witness, pure, 124; real, 123
witnessing Self, 130-131
work, 30, 110
Word, holy (God-into-expression), 9; commune with, 15; distinct from perishable regions, 66; true jnani communes with, 79; essence, 93; compared with Aum, 101-102; who communes with freed of Karmas, 104; for mor-

tals to listen to, 116; spirit force, God-in-action, 145; springs from Anaam, 146; they that have communed with shall have salvation, 159; pulls soul upward, 160; made flesh (guru), 160; related to Sraosha, 202; living master in constant touch with, 204; sowing in hearts of people, 206; came to John, 108, 207; in the beginning was the, 142, 209; as the living water, 210; masters have merged with, 212; was audible to Christ, 217; all-pervasiveness of, 222; personified (Saint), 224; manifestation of God's Will, 224; attunement with, 224; by communion with, 224; all in all, 226; given by the guru, 229; no evil influence can come near, 234; Divine stream radiating light and harmony, 236
wordless, 143, 146, 195, 199

Yajnas, 103, 118
Yajnavalkya, 4, 8
Yama, 102
Yamas and Niyamas, 24-30,* 28, 60, 84, 94, 197
Yeats, 149
Yog Nidra, 60, 77
Yoga, 4,* 20-23,* see Ashtang Yoga, Surat Shabd Yoga, Bhakti Yoga, etc., also Table of Contents
Yogendra, Shri, 94
yogi (yogin), 4, 66, 81, 93, 96, 98, 114, 120
yogishwara, 65, 93n., 115
Yoni, 37

Zarathustra, 202
Zikr, 29
Zoroaster, 101, 115, 116, 190, 202
Zoroastrianism, 143, 202-203*

OTHER BOOKS

BY KIRPAL SINGH

Godman: Finding a Spiritual Master
The Crown of Life: A Study in Yoga
Morning Talks
Naam or Word
Prayer: Its Nature and Technique
A Great Saint—Baba Jaimal Singh: His Life and Teachings
Jap Ji: The Message of Guru Nanak
Spiritual Elixir, Vols. I and II
The Teachings of Kirpal Singh (compiled and edited by Ruth Seader)
  Vol. I: The Holy Path
  Vol. II: Self-Introspection/Meditation
  Vol. III: The New Life (complete in one book)
Heart to Heart Talks—Vols. I and II (edited by Malcolm Tillis)
The Night Is a Jungle and Other Discourses of Kirpal Singh
Man! Know Thyself
Spirituality: What It Is
The Mystery of Death
The Wheel of Life: The Law of Action and Reaction
A Brief Life Sketch of Hazur Baba Sawan Singh Ji Maharaj
God Power, Christ Power, Guru Power

BY DARSHAN SINGH

Spiritual Awakening
The Secret of Secrets: Spiritual Talks
The Cry of the Soul: Mystic Poetry
Inner Space
The Meaning of Christ

BY OTHER AUTHORS

Portrait of Perfection: A Pictorial Biography of Kirpal Singh
The Beloved Master, edited by Bhadra Sena
Classics & Creations: A World of Vegetarian Cooking
The Ocean of Grace Divine, edited by Bhadra Sena
Seeing Is Above All: Sant Darshan Singh's First Indian Tour,
  edited by H.C. Chadda
Kirpal Singh: The Story of a Saint
  compiled and adapted for children; with illustrations

ORDERING BOOKS

Books listed on the preceding page may be ordered through your bookseller or directly from Sawan Kirpal Publications, Route 1, Box 24, Bowling Green, VA 22427, or Sawan Kirpal Publications, 2 Canal Road, Vijay Nagar, Delhi-110009, India.

SAT SANDESH: THE MESSAGE OF THE MASTERS

This monthly magazine is filled with practical and inspiring articles on all aspects of the mystic experience. Discourses by the living Master, Sant Darshan Singh, provide the initiate and seeker with information and guidance on meditation and the spiritual life. Also included are articles by Sant Kirpal Singh and Baba Sawan Singh. Poetry, photos, and other features appear in each issue. For subscription information write: Sat Sandesh, Subscription Dept., Route 1, Box 24, Bowling Green, VA 22427.

FURTHER INFORMATION

Mr. T.S. Khanna, General Representative, 8807 Lea Lane, Alexandria, VA 22309.

Olga Donenberg, Midwest Representative, 6007 N. Sheridan Rd., #14-B, Chicago, IL 60660.

Sunnie Cowen, Southern Representative, 3976 Belle Vista Dr. E, St. Petersburg Beach, FL 33706.

Sant Darshan Singh resides at Kirpal Ashram, 2 Canal Road, Vijay Nagar, Delhi-110009, India.